NARCISSISTIC FATHERS

AN EMOTIONAL *ABUSE*

WORKBOOK:

NARCISSISTIC STATES AND THE THERAPEUTIC PROCESS

by AMY LANDRY

CONTENTS

CHAPTER 1 - RECOGNIZE THE PROOLEM

Narcissism: What's this?

Narcissism is a rather overused term, representing a wide range of meanings, depending on whether it is used to describe a mental disorder, personality trait or general attitude inherent in today's culture.

In psychology, for pathological narcissism, we refer to the narcissistic personality disorder, which concerns all those subjects with a pathological egocentrism, in contact with an idealized and grandiose self-image, with an exaggerated sense of superiority fueled by fantasies of success, power and charm.

Narcissistic personality disorder includes egocentric and self-referenced behavior and thinking patterns, a total lack of empathy, little consideration of others, to which is added a deep need for admiration.

Narcissists defined as malignant or perverse (malignant narcissism and perverse narcissism) use manipulation and deception as a way of managing human relationships, behavior that often hides borderline, antisocial and paranoid personality traits.

This self-exaltation actually hides, as reported by DSM 5th edition (Diagnostic and Statistical Manual of Mental Disorders), deep feelings of insecurity, inadequacy and vulnerability to the judgment of others.

How to recognize it

Knowing how to recognize a pathological narcissist means paying attention to a series of warning signs, which can indicate that you are in front of a person who is highly disturbed and unable to build healthy and stable relationships.

Therefore, knowing the warning signs becomes of vital importance for the potential victims of those suffering from narcissistic personality disorder; such signs include:

Lack of empathy

Sense of arrogance - People with Narcissistic Personality Disorder expect special or exclusive treatment for them

Fantasies of grandeur and importance - Narcissists tend to surround themselves with people deemed worthy or through whom they can gain social prestige

Superficiality - People with narcissistic personality disorder are often very attached to their image and how it is perceived by others

Inability to manage and regulate their emotions in a healthy way - Narcissistic subjects tend to indulge in exaggerated reactions when something does not go as they had planned: in these cases, that is, when their needs for adoration and care are not satisfied, they show narcissistic anger

Hypersensitive to criticism - Despite the propensity to constant criticism of anyone around them, which often takes on the connotations of devaluation, narcissists are actually very fragile subjects and unable to manage criticism in an adult way; every slightest contradiction is experienced as a personal attack and de-legitimization of the false and grandiose self-image that they have built.

In the event that all six of these signs occur, it is good to be alert and try to get away as soon as possible from subjects who exhibit them.

ADDITIONAL CHARACTERISTICS OF THE NARCISSIST INCLUDE

The tendency to extreme jealousy

They practice what is called gaslighting, that is: through the manipulation they are capable of, they question the perception of the reality of those around them, making them doubt their own sanity. The denial of one's perception of reality can occur as follows: the narcissist's partner may for example say that he feels hurt by some action committed by the narcissist; the narcissist instead of admitting to having hurt the partner or listening to him and trying to clarify the situation, will deny that the partner has felt hurt or will deny having said the words that actually hurt the partner; in this way, the victim of the narcissist will question himself and his perception of reality; that's why in these cases it becomes important to record the conversations

- Little loyalty to partner or to any relationship

- Being subject to frequent outbursts.

Symptoms

Symptoms of pathological narcissism include:

- Exaggerated sense of superiority
- Unlimited success, power and fascination fantasies
- Hypersensitivity to criticism and failure
- Sense of emptiness and apathy despite successes
- Need to be admired

Lack of empathy

Deep sense of vulnerability, insecurity and fragility, never managed in a healthy way.

To these symptoms is often added the abuse of substances (such as alcohol and / or drugs), taken in an attempt to put an end to the restlessness, typical of this pathology.

Causes

Narcissistic personality disorder, like many other psychopathological disorders, seems to be caused by the mixture of several factors, hereditary and environmental, which contribute to its development.

Several studies argue that the cause of narcissism is to be found in early experiences that are not very reassuring with attachment figures, due to which the subject would react with a strong emotional disinvestment towards the other and turning his attention towards himself or, again, parenting attitudes that encourage and reward a grandiose image of the child's self.

Another hypothesis accredited by several researchers is that the child is (or has been) the victim of bullying and humiliation, especially by peers, and could, as a consequence, try to overcome this continuous attack on his self-esteem by a great sense of self.

TREATMENT OF NARCISSISM

The request for treatment that narcissists make to a specialist, a psychologist or psychotherapist, is rarely aimed at the resolution of the narcissistic disorder: these subjects, in fact, cannot conceive of being able to have serious relational or personality dysfunctions.

Usually, a subject suffering from narcissistic personality disorder turns to these figures in an attempt to resolve or stem some secondary manifestations, therefore panic attacks or depressive states, which arise from the fact that the feared representation of self (that of a failed self and anything but great) has entered their consciousness.

Among the treatments for narcissism considered most effective for the cure we can mention:

Cognitive Behavioral Therapy - Its goal is to replace dysfunctional automatic thoughts with more adaptive and realistic ones using the technique of cognitive restructuring;

Drug therapy - Drug treatment usually includes SSRIs or selective serotonin reuptake inhibitors, anticonvulsant drugs and mood stabilizers that address: anxiety, social anxiety, hypochondria, depression and rabid helplessness, symptoms that most of the time they motivate the request for help.

What to do

When approaching a pathological narcissist, one must bear in mind that they are fragile individuals, in need of attention, affection and admiration, who have unwittingly built a grandiose image of themselves as a defensive barrier.

For anyone living with a narcissist it is good to learn to accept their limitations. Claiming support or attention from a person with narcissism often has a counterproductive effect that leads the narcissist to increase his requests for attention and care even more, since he is unable to give it.

When dealing with a narcissistic person, don't seek their approval. Pleasing a narcissus is, most of the time, an impossible mission, this is because the excessive ego leads them to consider others as inferior and, therefore, civilizable in every respect.

It is advisable to avoid taking their utterances seriously and seek professional help if the emotional burden of a relationship with a narcissist is too heavy to carry on your own.

HOW TO DEFEND YOURSELF

The people who most need to defend themselves against a narcissist are those who know them well: family members, partners, friends, and co-workers.

Often, people who enter into a relationship with the narcissist and are emotionally damaged by it have some characteristics that fall within the psychological condition known as affective codependency.

People who often end up entangled in relationships with a narcissist, also known as victims, have the following psychological characteristics:

Tendency to complacency and submission - Typical of a person who accepts any request and has a hard time saying no

Low assertiveness - That is, having difficulty expressing one's opinion to others

Low self-esteem

Sense of inadequacy

Being used to criticism in relationships, from childhood

High sense of sacrifice.

So, if you review these characteristics and suspect you are in a relationship with a person with *Narcissistic Personality Disorder*, here's what to do: first of all, it is necessary to interrupt the relationship; then you will need all the help you can, trusted friends and relatives who may be able to understand the situation but above all a professional in psychology.

Thanks to psychological therapy, it is in fact possible to begin to work on oneself and on what has determined a strong attachment to a dysfunctional relationship. Finally, here are some things that you will need to work on thanks to your therapist to recover from the abuse that the narcissist has inflicted on a psychological level:

Working on your self-esteem - Reflecting and recognizing your own worth will progressively prevent someone from trying to belittle or mock your abilities and therefore humiliate as an insidious tool of manipulation.

Staying autonomous - Establishing emotional and physical boundaries in which to exercise one's well-being is essential for creating healthy relationships. Being autonomous or being able to take care of oneself, one's own economic resources and one's passions and interests without interference is important not only for one's own well-being, but also to prevent a possible narcissist from trying to direct all the efforts of the other on oneself and on the satisfaction of one's needs.

Exercising assertiveness - Practicing expressing one's opinion is critical to affirming one's self-esteem and uniqueness, which the narcissist wants to erode and then be able to better manipulate the victim.

FEMALE NARCISSISM

Statistically 75% of individuals with narcissistic personality disorder are men, yet in recent years we are witnessing a drastic increase in cases of female narcissism.

Narcissistic women are charming people, dedicated to self-care and career, but unlike men they are not avoidant, selfish or unaffectionate; indeed, often, it is a question of women who almost obsessively dedicate themselves to a couple relationship or family life.

Other characteristics of female narcissism usually include:

- Excessive emotionality
- Self-indulgence and inability to take responsibility for one's mistakes
- Persistent manipulation of the other to achieve one's goals.

The point in common with male narcissism is the avoidance of intimacy: the narcissistic woman does not want and cannot show herself fragile, she cannot risk compromising herself in the authentic relationship with the other; for this, the other must become perfect as she requires: a practically impossible undertaking.

WHAT GOES THROUGH THE MIND OF A NARCISSIST?

Often people are not exactly what they appear to us. Except when we lie deliberately, when we behave in ways that do not reflect our feelings, emotions, thoughts, there can be infinite reasons and situations in which what appears on the outside does not exactly match what we feel inside. It happens for us, just as it happens for the people around us.

Every human being is a real mystery in the eyes of others, and in many cases even in front of himself. Sometimes unconscious or subconscious reasons can cause us to say, think, or act in completely unexpected and unpredictable ways.

In the case of a person with strong narcissistic traits, appearances are not always able to faithfully portray how a person feels deep down. In the face of a bold, self-confident person with a strong personality, in many cases there is an individual with low self-esteem, fragile, unstable.

Mostly they are accused of loving only themselves, in reality they can come to harbor immense contempt for themselves. Self-flattery, perfectionism, arrogance are part of a larger mask that if it falls could reveal an image of themselves that they believe can be devastating. Their search for social validation, for continuous external confirmations and gratifications represents a fallacious attempt to fill themselves with that love that they themselves are unable to grant to themselves or to give to others.

What is Narcissistic Personality Disorder?

In order to speak of Narcissistic Personality Disorder, the person must exhibit at least 5 of the following traits:

- display an exaggerated sense of self-importance, one's achievements and talents
- dreaming of power, success, brilliance, limitless beauty or ideal love
- believe yourself to be special, unique, to be understood or to be associated exclusively with other equally special or high-status people
- require an excess of admiration
- expect favorable treatment, condescension to one's wishes, without particular reason
- exploit and take advantage of others to achieve their goals
- not being empathetic towards the emotions, feelings, needs of others
- envy others or believe that you are envied by them
- having arrogant attitudes or behaviors.

In fact, according to psychiatrist James F. Masterson, there are two types of narcissism: exhibitionistic and covert. The first tends to magnify himself and denigrate the other when he does not recognize him as such, the second, on the other hand, shows low self-esteem, denigrates himself, is ashamed, refuses, humiliates himself, feels a strong sense of emptiness.

HOW NARCISSISM ARISES

Sometimes it can be very difficult to understand and empathize with a person with strong narcissistic traits. However, such people did not deliberately choose to become that. In large part it is assumed that their way of being must be attributed to a developmental arrest that was caused by a parental deficiency in which the reference figure (maternal or not) did not provide sufficient nourishment or was very indulgent, or very harsh and critical. Other theories, however, hypothesize a genetic cause in the onset of this disorder.

In the case of exhibitionistic narcissism, the parental figures have helped to make the child feel exceptional, better than others, have covered him with unrealistic expectations of success, that everything is due, without giving anything in return, that everything is lawful. This arouses self-indulgent, aggressive, intolerant, self-centered behavior, lacking collaboration, cooperation and healthy emotional relationships.

The case of hidden narcissism, on the other hand, occurs when the parental figure lacks recognition, acceptance, and care for the child. The sense of inferiority, of non-acceptance, of self-depreciation, of shame, of inferiority that derives from it can lead to creating a special, different self-image as compensation for a self-value that has been denied and disowned.

HOW A NARCISSIST RELATES

People with strong narcissistic traits tend to behave very differently in public and in private. In the latter context they can come to dispute and strongly denigrate those around them. With loved ones and even more in a couple relationship, after a brief initial idyll, the expectations of being recognized, appreciated, flattered by virtue of their presumed being special for various reasons begin to manifest.

They can try to achieve this through criticism, denigrating the other, in order not to bring out and defend themselves from their own tendency to shame and self-humiliation. In this way they tend to make the relationship revolve around their person and perceive the partner as an extension of themselves.

Many narcissists are perfectionists. They believe that what others say, do or are is never good or never good enough. They expect the partner to respond unconditionally to any of their needs, especially in terms of acceptance, appreciation, service, love, and when this does not happen, they feel rejected.

They cannot accept "no", and often expect the other to respond to their needs, even without declaring them openly. They tend to manipulate the other, make him feel guilty, punish him if he doesn't behave as they expect.

Trying to meet the demands and expectations of a person with strong narcissistic traits is an almost endless effort. They manage to make the other's efforts feel in vain, or they praise him in a purely formal way. Even when they seem to be finally satisfied, they quickly return to scorn, denigrate, or ask for even more.

The partner perceives them as cold, distant, unavailable. The emotional deprivation they experienced as a child makes them dependent on others, insatiable and continually in search of nourishment, satisfaction, recognition by others.

Over time the partner begins to question them, what their true personality is, if they are truly manipulative individuals or if it is a mask they wear. They constantly feel attacked, criticized, emptied, exhausted by behavior bordering on the unpredictable.

They end up neglecting other relationships and bonds, as well as their personal interests in order to get absorbed by the needs of the partner. They are constantly squeezed between the risks of devaluation, attack, quarrels, strong expressions of affection and the sudden breakdown of the relationship.

Over time, the partner of a highly narcissistic person learns to live with a partner who is cold and unwilling to abandon himself emotionally. In the long run they begin to doubt themselves, they lose confidence and self-esteem. Even if these experiences are shared with the narcissistic partner, he becomes defensive.

Despite these difficulties, the partner tends to remain in the relationship because the periodic manifestations of affection, emotionality, excitement, love, passion can partially counterbalance the moments of coldness, detachment, criticism, attack. Such episodes typically occur when the narcissist feels that the breakup of the relationship is imminent.

When both partners have strong traits of narcissism it is an open struggle to make their desires, needs, needs prevail and punish each other when the other does not seem to respect their needs.

Narcissists tend to keep their distance within a relationship, even more so when there is sexual closeness. They want to keep control and power. The idea of being dependent is inconceivable, because it makes them feel weak, fragile and above all exposes them to the risk of rejection and shame. In turn, the partner tends to chase them, because in fact, underneath, both partners feel unlovable and the risk of emotional abandonment would be a replica of what they have experienced in the past.

10 TYPES OF NARCISSISM: THE DIFFERENT FACES OF NARCISSISTIC PEOPLE

People with narcissistic personality disorder develop a deeply self-centered attitude, believing that they are of vital importance to everyone. They don't have enough mental flexibility to realize that we are all important to some and insignificant to others.

Characteristics of narcissistic people

The narcissistic personality is characterized by:

- Feelings of grandeur and arrogance. The narcissistic person often exaggerates their accomplishments and talents, usually with the goal of having others

recognize and praise them, even if they are not actually successful.
- She suffers from fantasies of success, power, brilliance or beauty that have no confirmation in reality, which leads her to live in a sort of "alternative world" where everything is perfect.
- Exploits interpersonal relationships, uses others to achieve their goals or satisfy their needs.
- Lacks empathy, is not willing to recognize or identify with the feelings and needs of others.
- She believes that others envy her for her alleged achievements or talents.

Types of narcissism

Generally speaking, three main types of narcissism can be referred to, based on how one seeks admiration and attention:

- Exhibitionist narcissist, who needs the admiration of others and, for this, does not hesitate to exaggerate or invent his successes and / or talents.
- Introverted narcissist, who seeks the attention of others by assuming the role of the victim, through subtle manipulation strategies.
- Toxic narcissist, who satisfies his needs for admiration through control, power and harassment, making others feel inferior.

These types of narcissism develop into more specific personological profiles:

Emotional addicted narcissist

He simply believes he doesn't have enough love, feels slightly dissatisfied with the attention of others, but experiences a void of approval and affection. Underlying this behavior is a deep fear of rejection and abandonment, so the narcissist clings to the addiction.

To meet these needs, he has no qualms about manipulating others. His emotional demands are on the rise, so his partner and those close to him are emotionally drained to try to nurture, comfort and support that "me" that is so in need of affection.

Tyrant narcissist

This type of narcissism ties into power because it has an insatiable need for domination and authority. This person behaves arrogantly, believes he is superior, often despises others and treats them as if they are "inferior". He thinks he is always right and in control of the situation, so his mere presence is often overwhelming. When such a narcissist takes control, he makes life impossible for his subordinates. When he's in a relationship, he uses it as a trophy. He generally denigrates people, who are simply a means of demonstrating his power and satisfying his need for authority.

Elite narcissist

In order for others to know and pay homage to him, he never tires of proclaiming his supposed successes and achievements. He usually exaggerates his importance because he wants to arouse envy or admiration. This narcissistic person always offers his opinion, even when it is not asked for, and thinks he knows more than anyone else, regardless of the subject in question. He often thinks he is destined to do great things and deserves great things, but does nothing to make them happen. Often, he is a charismatic person, in such a way that he manages to attract many followers into his "orbit", who eventually realize that "it's all smoke but no fire".

Imaginative narcissist

This narcissistic person develops very elaborate fantasies, to the point that almost his entire life is spent in his inner world. When this person relates to others, he shows his inner world as if it were real, so he lies repeatedly. A fictitious life is usually invented to arouse the envy and admiration of others. And he doesn't recognize his lies, even when put face to face with reality, he's always looking for an excuse to keep his fantasies standing.

Somatic narcissist

Feeling good and being fit is important for health, but this type of narcissism goes a step further, because it is an obsession with the body and beauty. This person's scale of values comes down to image, fashion, beauty, youth, and glamor. She needs to be admired for her physical characteristics and her self-esteem is inextricably linked to her body image. This narcissistic person is usually a perfectionist and takes a long time over her body and beauty care rituals. The problem is that she applies this pattern to others as well and judges them by their physical appearance. She also thinks she deserves everything due to her beauty and fitness.

Antagonist narcissist

This is a fairly common type of narcissism in which anger simmers beneath the surface. Unhappiness manifests itself in growing hostility towards everyone. Often experiences episodes of explosive anger with "irrational", disconcerting or inexplicable causes. Usually he resorts to verbal violence, insults, with his words, those close to him causing them a lot of damage. Hypersensitivity hides behind this behavior, so when this person does not receive the praise and admiration he expected, he can come to interpret any word as an insult or disrespect. He assumes everything as if it were a personal attack, and that causes his anger. The involvement of the "I" is called a narcissistic injury.

Cheating narcissist

This type of narcissism shows its best side. The person is charming, attractive and friendly. At least in the beginning. Unfortunately, this attraction is just a mask that hides a much murkier personality. Behind the "trust me" messages hide malicious intentions. In reality, the narcissist wants to gain the trust of others to use it in his favor. He practices a kind of "emotional vandalism" where the damage is so terrible that victims often take years to recover and trust someone else. This narcissist uses his charm-to-charm others and give them their energy.

Martyr narcissist

This narcissist's personal identity is built around grief, being a victim or even a survivor. Suffering justifies his need for attention and the parasitic demands that result in unbalanced relationships brought about by exploitation. Obviously, this person carries huge emotional baggage. The pain of the past never goes away. He pollutes the present with this suffering which, in his mind, makes him an exceptional person. Interacting with this type of narcissist can become very complicated because he never meets the needs of support that we all need, but constantly demands support and attention for himself, because no one has suffered more than him. When he is denied such attention, he will not hesitate to hurl accusations to generate a sense of guilt that allows him to remain a martyr.

Messianic narcissist

This type of narcissism is based on a "high moral ground." They are narcissistic people who see themselves as more helpful, good and kind than others, so they often look down on others and criticize them. He will present himself as a savior, but in reality, his seemingly selfless help includes many implicit conditions. This person will not hesitate to claim favors and ask for constant praise for his alleged "sacrifice", so the relationship turns into a permanent debt.

Vengeful narcissist

He has no qualms about creating conflicts in his path or making up lies about his competitors. He can do anything to bring down his "enemies". Instead of trying to grow and improve, this narcissist suffers from Procrustean Syndrome and despises all those who excel, so he tries to frame and defame them to damage their reputation. In this way he can return to the center of attention and admiration.

The narcissistic person needs psychological help because deep self-centeredness harms those around him and generates unhappiness. These are just a few tips on how to deal with a narcissist without losing your psychological balance.

THE PSYCHOLOGICAL PROFILE OF A MANIPULATIVE NARCISSIST

When we talk about manipulation, we mean the ability to influence a person's decisions and choices, inducing him to adopt behaviors, which most likely did not choose to act freely, through the use of seduction and leveraging his sensitivity and vulnerability. Every manipulation is a more or less explicit aggression, whoever is subject to it recognizes himself as he loses the ability to oppose decisions made by the manipulator, to reflect and to choose in full autonomy.

The paradox of a relationship with a manipulative narcissist is that the victim, while recognizing the abuse he is undergoing, presents enormous difficulties in getting rid of it. The relationship between the manipulative narcissist and his victim is determined by the fact that both are marked by early relational traumatic experiences to which they have reacted differently, making it seemingly impossible to react to the seduction, the sense of guilt and the false promises that the victim suffers. It is essential to remember that the manipulative narcissist can be both a man or a woman, by convention in this chapter we will use the male gender when talking about a manipulative narcissist but it is always useful to remember that it is a mode of behavior that can be found in both genders.

What are the elements that allow you to recognize a manipulative narcissist?

In order to identify a manipulative narcissist, it is essential to recognize some of his peculiar characteristics including:

- Reactions amplified with respect to any situation that causes annoyance to the point of causing violent behavior.
- He appears lovable and polite in public while in private he shows aggression, violence and verbal and physical devaluation.
- His reactions are unpredictable as it is not possible to understand what and when it can be annoying, so his presence generates a continuous state of alertness and tension in those around him.
- He does not take responsibility and when he makes mistakes, he attributes the mistakes to others.
- He is very clear about the goals he wants to achieve and how to achieve them.
- His point of view is unique and indisputable and in order to keep it that way he questions and does not accept the opinions of others even if motivated.

It resorts to blackmail directly or indirectly.

He is not clear in expressing his opinions and expects others to understand them as if they had to resort to reading his thoughts. He changes his mind when he realizes that it is no longer useful in achieving his goals.

Depending on the situation it changes opinions and behaviors in an opportunistic way.

He does not get involved and exploits people to express his ideas.

He is very fickle but does not accept that others can be too.

He is permissive with himself but rigid and intolerant with close people towards whom he does not tolerate mistakes as he expects them to be perfect.

He is critical of everything and all people by questioning the skills and competency of others.

He is insecure, he prefers to always be with the same people and the same environments since moving away from known models and relationships does not allow him to control them.

He belittles and devalues others to compensate for his insecurity.

He befriends ignorant and incompetent people to emphasize his superiority.

He uses friends, family and couple relationships for his own personal gain.

He doesn't listen and tells lies.

He interprets reality to obtain his own advantage.

He controls and limits the freedom of choice of the people with whom he comes into contact and has a relationship.

He passes himself off as a victim when he needs the compassion of others.

Are manipulative narcissists all the same or are there different types?

The dominator and the despotic: he is recognized because he is an arrogant and despotic person, he criticizes everyone and is characterized by an authoritarian attitude. He humiliates the people he relates to until they no longer expose themselves for fear of his reactions. He is sure that his point of view is unique and absolute, he has no regard for the moods and lives of others. He does not respect the rules that apply to others but not to him.

The likeable: he's a person able to hold a pleasant conversation, wants to be the center of attention and uses manipulation by resorting to joke and irony to embarrass the people around him.

The low profile: he is the typical person who appears unable to resolve situations and who delegates their resolution to others. He never exposes himself and tries to push others to do something he knows to be unfair or dangerous.

The prophet: he believes he can predict what will happen despite not having real elements on which to base this forecast, he does not accept elements of reality other than those he takes into consideration. He has a high opinion of himself to avoid adapting and considering the decisions of others.

The seducer: is distinguished by physical attractiveness and pleasant and charming ways, sometimes for good social position and profession. He uses his charm to manipulate others to adhere to his demands.

The generous: he is an apparent altruist, available to everyone without ever asking for anything. The problem arises when he expects his actions to be reciprocated as he has acted in an apparently disinterested way, developing expectations of reciprocity. The victim of the generous manipulative narcissist will find it very difficult to free himself as it will not be easy to stem the sense of guilt induced by the duty to reciprocate.

The cultured: he is a storyteller and monopolizes the conversation to impress others. He leverages the ignorance of others to strengthen his own image as a cultured person and does not hesitate to exhibit the qualifications and knowledge in order to humiliate the other. At the base there is always a deep insecurity and a low self-esteem.

The explosive: he manifests significant reactions of anger as he accumulates within himself emotions and sensations that are stratified and become unsustainable when he is faced with situations that are unsustainable for him. Anxiety, fear, a sense of inferiority, push him to look for a scapegoat on which to let off steam without then apologizing.

The helpless: They pretend to be weak and helpless, in need of help and expect others to take care of him and fix the mistakes he has made due to lack of responsibility in making his own choices.

The employee: uses others as an appendage of himself, imagining that they are always at his disposal to satisfy his requests and expects the other to understand his needs and to approach him.

The sick person: during childhood or adolescence he experienced a condition of illness of which he understood the secondary advantages to keep the family members connected to him in a state of apprehension. As an adult, he always uses his state of health to attract attention and to maintain control over the actions and decisions of others, generating feelings of guilt in those close to him in such a way as to never feel abandoned

The sowers of discord: They spend their time figuring out how to achieve their results through lying and generating discord among the people they know. Usually, this type of manipulation occurs mainly among women.

The perverse: he never feels guilt and treats people as objects. He feels the need to belittle in order to increase his self-esteem. He needs admiration and approval, and to achieve them he has no respect for those around him.

To fully understand the personality of the manipulative narcissist, we are helped by the words of the psychoanalyst O. Kernberg who, in the work "Marginal syndromes and pathological narcissism" defines them as "people who have a great need to be loved and admired and who hide the contradiction between a very inflated and boundless opinion of oneself that needs to receive the tribute of others.

Their emotional life lacks depth; they have little sympathy for the feelings of others and little reason to enjoy life, they envy others; they tend to idealize certain individuals and belittle others.

In general, their relationships have the clear purpose of exploiting others and sometimes of becoming real parasites. It is as if they feel the right to control and possess others and exploit them without any sense of guilt. Under their apparent sympathy and charm it is possible to perceive a cold and merciless nature".

What is the psychological profile of the manipulative narcissist?

The manipulative narcissist, while appearing to be a safe and solid person, actually has little self-confidence and feels very fragile, uses manipulative behavior, sometimes unconsciously and others less so, to defend himself from the deep sense of anguish and insecurity that pervades. Manipulation is an automatic process that is structured during the evolutionary process, a real means of survival, if he did not resort to it, he would be devoured by anguish and fear.

Most likely he was exposed to a model of manipulative behavior from an early age during which he was not taken into consideration emotionally feeling excluded, so he had to find a way to attract attention. The manipulatory model of reference is usually one of the most significant and important affective figures, for which the manipulation mechanism implemented as an adult allows him to appear to control the thoughts and feelings of people dear to him or who have something important, in his eyes. The deepest personal feelings of the manipulative narcissist are characterized by a strong dose of anger that is systematically repressed, so that it becomes an emotional charge that comes out in the most unexpected moments.

The paradox of this condition is that the desire for control will never allow him to fill the sense of emptiness and insecurity it brings with it. It is inconceivable for this type of personality to accept the idea that people have desires independent of his own, as if it were irreconcilable the idea that wishes that are not his own can coexist as they would risk the annihilation of his person and his own desire, deemed unique.

Probably this personality structure has its roots in the mother's inability to decode her child's needs, perceived as a threat and an obstacle to satisfying her own desires. The effect of this vision of reality has led the mother to imagine that her desire and that of the child cannot coexist because if it satisfies that of the child, she cannot fulfill her own, so an open conflict is generated to see which of the two can triumph. Such a mother is a person who is unable to decode the language and the needs of the child who remain unsatisfied due to misinterpretations and self-referencing. According to the psychologist Laura Gutman the emotional violence that is perpetuated by the mother against the child consists in the impossibility that the desires of both can coexist in the same emotional field, this experience is the same that the manipulator brings with him to adult life and continues to perpetuate.

According to this logic, the desire of the other is a threat to his own, according to his experiences he should step aside but this is not possible for him because the manipulator wants everything for fear of having nothing. He constantly feels in danger of emotional life and lives a continuous state of alert as every confrontation is experienced as a conflict from which he must emerge victorious in order not to feel annihilated. Any desire other than his own is an invasion and dangerous for his own existence, so the manipulator wants to control the thoughts and actions of anyone he deems threatening because he has different desires from his own.

He feels he has to destroy the enemy if his emotional existence is in jeopardy, so he resorts to all kinds of manipulations to survive this fear. The manipulative narcissist has the presumption that he knows everything and does not accept alternative ideas to his own, he is unable to share anything since there is only room for his desires.

The manipulative narcissist is recognized for some distinctive traits including that of avoiding giving information about himself while being very curious to know the details of the lives of others as in this way he imagines having more power and hiding his own insecurity. By blaming and devaluing others, he deludes himself to increase the level of his own self-esteem, he attributes to others all the aspects he detests about himself through a massive use of projection. He perceives the victim as an impending danger from which he must protect himself and attack before they carry out an evil deed (fruit of the projection of the narcissist).

The strategies he uses are those of belittling and discrediting the opponent and generating a sense of guilt in him. The victim will try in every way to give his reasons but it will not help as the attack of the manipulative narcissist will be incessant so a spiral is created in which the manipulative narcissist attacks, the victim tries to explain and the narcissist devalues and generates senses of guilt. This whole process is then permeated by lies and misunderstandings that the narcissist carries out to his own advantage, often resorting to silence in order to never expose himself and always leave a loophole open. These behaviors have the effect on the victim of generating doubts, destabilizing and confusing, to the point of pushing them to make decisions against their will. Finally, the manipulative narcissist often avoids direct confrontation because by constantly changing his opinion, he never wants to take responsibility for his actions and confuses his victims in every way, sending conflicting messages to put them in the condition that whatever the victim does will always be wrong or it will never be enough.

NARCISSISTIC PARENTS: WHEN THE NARCISSIST IS MOM OR DAD

We often talk about narcissism and toxic relational dynamics in the couple relationship, but we often forget to analyze how these relational dynamics affect children.

In fact, the affective and relational dynamics are internalized by the children in the form of "scripts", relationship patterns, attachment styles and have a positive or negative impact on their emotional life.

Each of us can easily realize how certain fears, behavior patterns, sensations, emotions "trigger automatically" work as a "compulsion to repeat" of familiar scripts already experienced.

It is not enough to realize that what we experienced in the family is wrong, made us suffer and that we do not want to reactivate it to be safe; these patterns are unconscious, atavistic and are triggered in every situation that reactivates that emotional and behavioral pattern, especially when we find ourselves embodying the role of the husband / wife or parent and for this unconsciously identifying with the abusive parent (both from a point of physical or emotional view) is easy.

Why does it happen?

Because in nature a puppy tends to imitate those behaviors that guarantee its survival, for this reason - often - it is psychologically easier to identify with the aggressor than with the victim.

In the most complex cases the entire sado-masochistic relationship pattern is internalized and therefore the roles of victim and executioner in adult relationships alternate.

For a parent who is psychologically and emotionally immature - which we generically define as "narcissist" - but who could belong to various personality styles connected to narcissism (histrionic, border, paranoid ..), children are projections of their ego, they are trophies, objects that they must directly or indirectly satisfy or repay them for the fatigue caused or for the desires of realization that they did not have the courage to pursue or for which they failed; even worse, the children are those who will have to redeem their emotional wound, take part in feuds of family revenge or take care of them by repaying everything given to them (often little to nothing on an emotional level but a lot on a material level).

An immature parent relates to his child as if he were already grown up, rejects his affective and emotional needs, especially those concerning the processes of emotional self-regulation; then the child is praised if he wins, if he is good, if he makes us look good, if he is a mirror that reflects an idealized image of the parent, but when he shows negative parts of himself, he is devalued, criticized, rejected or humiliated.

This happens because an emotionally immature parent is unable to tolerate his negative parts and process them, so when an emotional commitment is required, he gets scared and projects all his failures or deficiencies onto others.

For a narcissist there are no spots or faults, a narcissist does not take on emotional responsibilities; in front of them he runs away or humiliates you because you have them and you are weak.

It is always someone else's fault and if he admits the fault it is because he had to react like that because of someone else.

You are unfortunate if that "someone else" is you, but often, in this type of dysfunctional pattern, the narcissist (especially if it works at a border level) alternates the figure of the persecutor with that of the victim or the angry child with both the partner, that with the children... as if to say the scenario often changes victim in turn.

What happens is the intergenerational transmission of abusive emotional and reactive dynamics and / or repressive educational styles based on the victim-executioner dyad, in which the victim of today is often the persecutor of tomorrow (role reversal).

When a parent is perceived as untrustworthy, he alternates moments of availability with others in which he is aggressive, terrifying or he devalues and humiliates them. What occurs is a complete dissociation from the disturbing emotional aspects connected to these experiences (affective avoidance) and / or the development of a disorganized or anxious attachment style (avoidant insecure / ambivalent insecure.

The ambivalence is given by the conflict that the child develops towards this type of parent: on the one hand he / she loves us, on the other hand he humiliates us and despises us or in the worst case hurts us. It is a paradox.

Furthermore, if you are a child, defenseless and still totally dependent you CANNOT CHOOSE and you are forced to stay there until you have the means to be INDEPENDENT by developing more or less consciously psychological defense and reaction strategies.

All this gives rise to a very strong ANGER which is often DISSOCIATED from the conscience, that is, the person does not realize that he feels it.

Emotionally dissociating is an inevitable strategy to keep the parent figure intact and save it from complete disintegration, while avoiding the psychic disintegration itself.

In years in the clinic, I have seen many people report terrifying emotional experiences or describe abuses (even severe physical ones) laughing and subsequently justifying their parents in the name of a sense of family or socio-cultural idealisms regarding self-sacrifice (children must be grateful, they have to understand, it wasn't easy for them, it's my fault ...)

Yes, because the paradox of the traumas of psychological abuse is also this, the guilt is almost always internalized by the victim.

An invisible guilt, for existing, for being born, for having an emotional need, for getting dirty, for not being perfect ...

Any detail (even useless) can be, for the narcissistic parent, a trigger of intolerance, anger and therefore of devaluation, humiliation or in the worst cases physical aggression.

The will of the children is not contemplated, they must satisfy parental expectations, sacrificing their ego, as Winnicott said, their true self at the expense of a false complacent self.

How to tell if our parents were emotionally immature?

It acts through emotional or moral blackmail: if you do this you don't love mom, if you talk to that person you hurt mom / dad, if you choose that school you disappoint dad, if you cry Jesus gets angry and you will go to hell ... You can't do this to me...

This adultizes the child by using it as a substitute for the partner: the parent takes out the quarrels he has with his partner with the child, asks him for moral or emotional support or even worse, asks him to hate the other parent because he / she made him / her suffer, or financial abuse (you have to contribute for the family because it is your duty ... too bad that it is often parents who do not work and make excuses for not cannibalizing their children!).

The narcissist is addicted to children but in conflict with this addiction and generates anxiety in them: the immature parent makes the children feel special by often telling them that without them he could not live, that they are unique and defending them at the sword with the outside world, but within the four walls he complains of them as if they were sores or condemnations attacking them psychologically and often physically, (affective ambivalence).

A narcissistic / emotionally immature parent often offers economic advantages to the child to keep him in a blackmailing state of addiction: "if you study engineering, instead of economics, dad will share the family business ... on the contrary, leave the house".

It devalues and humiliates any initiative of the child on a professional level: "but what are you doing, you are useless ... you are not capable, you make people laugh, that is not a job."

He threatens his children that he will no longer love them if they go away from home and prevents this from happening with all his might. "As long as you stay here, do what I tell you, if you go away you are no longer my son / daughter, I will close your accounts, I will take away any property ..."

He has deep fits of anger and aggression when the child puts an emotional or psychological or even physical boundary (he goes to live elsewhere for example).

Drag the child into marital or personal conflicts by using him as a shield or tool.

He is interested in controlling his son, using his power and not seeing him happy: "that is not the woman for you, you have to choose a woman who knows how to cook, make x or y, someone like your mother ..."

He is emotionally nourished by his son, who is often appointed to act as his handmaid / servant threatened by moral guilt: "Would you leave the family now that mother is sick"?

He uses his children as a punchbag to let off steam when he is nervous

He is often a perfectionist about goals to pursue, earnings, career and transfers very strong performance anxiety to his children

He is not empathetic and often seems to feel no remorse or guilt

Child abuse. He does not deal with the negative emotions of children, and when the children manifest them, he attacks or laughs at them so that they show strength, reactivity and do not show themselves weak, because for narcissists, VULNERABILITY is a huge threat.

In the most serious cases PHYSICALLY OR
SEXUALLY ABUSE OF CHILDREN:
Remember that IT IS NOT YOUR FAULT.
THERE IS NO SITUATION THAT CAN JUSTIFY
EMOTIONAL OR PHYSICAL ABUSE!!!

THEY ARE THE WEAK ONES.

NOT YOU.

And how is it done then? Can we solve this situation on our own?

NO, IT IS IMPOSSIBLE WITHOUT
KNOWLEDGE AND TOOLS AND WITHOUT
THEIR COLLABORATION.

Narcissists do not possess the communication and relational skills necessary to communicate on an emotional / affective level and also on a cognitive level. They DISTORT ANY REALITY IN THEIR FAVOR. These people don't really listen and abuse their psychological and material power.

What developmental trajectories are expected for the children?

Generally, these abuses lead (at different levels of severity) to post-traumatic personalities (from personality style to disorder) in which there are very specific relationship patterns that concern mistrust / abuse, abandonment, pessimism, self-sacrifice, submission, the pursuit of attention, the inability to self-control, failure, claims of grandeur, shame and social isolation.

Dependent or counter-dependent personalities: these personalities are characterized by a strong tendency to negativity, pessimism, insecurity, low self-esteem and from an emotional point of view very strong abandonment fears are common that prevent them from realizing themselves and their own personality.

Here then are depression, self-destructive and self-sabotaging behaviors both on the working and emotional level (search for partners who directly or indirectly remind him of the parent).

On the emotional level, these disappointed children, now adults, will seek the constant presence of a partner, (fears of abandonment) often abusive, in which they will act as victims or as passive-aggressive, in the case of counter-dependence they will show themselves avoiding and detached, disinterested with respect to ties, denying their own emotional and affective needs, experienced as a fragility to be ashamed of.

Development of a Borderline Personality: "Individuals with borderline personality disorder exhibit marked emotional instability, can experience moments of tranquility and quickly feel strong sadness, anger or guilt. Sometimes they experience a strong emotional chaos given by experiencing conflicting emotions at the same time. Regulating their emotional states is difficult and they often act impulsively, without reflecting on the consequences of their actions. They are accompanied by feelings of abandonment, often associated with an inability to be alone and the dire need to have a person with them.

The perception of separation / loss and rejection can lead to even profound alterations of self-image, mood, cognitive processes and behavior.

People with borderline personality disorder often tend to idealize other people and quickly devalue them, feeling that the other person in question does not care enough for them or is not "present" enough.

Individuals with BPD exhibit recurrent suicidal behaviors, gestures or threats, or self-injurious behaviors.

They may have a boycott pattern of themselves when the goal is on the verge of being fulfilled (e.g. drop out of school when they're close to graduation). Some individuals may develop psychotic-like symptoms (eg hallucinations) during periods of high stress. "

Development of a Histrionic, Paranoid or Narcissistic personality: these former abused children soon realize that nobody can be trusted, not even their parents, and that receiving attention, manipulating others, yields many advantages, which is why they try to make their sufferings, or to redeem them by becoming their "bullies", "the stars", "the smart ones", pursuing high goals, which detach them both materially and emotionally from family and society.

These masks of grandeur often act as protective shields or indirect devaluations towards parents or the outside world. "I am better than them". Everything that exists that is not free must be conquered and deserved, for if I do not get this / that I am a failure. "I don't even trust my mother, never mind you!"

Unconsciously they enter into love relationships with the desire to destroy the other, especially if this other really loves them.

The professional choice can be directed towards professions that guarantee social prestige (artists for example) or economic, political (positions of power) or moral (helping professions that imply strong tendencies towards self-sacrifice and self-denial for the other, but also great search for human gratitude).

The search for these important positions is so intense that it often does not include the possibility of living or being happy and sometimes the goals these people achieve are not even what they would have liked.

From an emotional point of view, these people identify with the aggressor and therefore show themselves cynical, contemptuous, poorly empathetic and very aggressive.

They also suffer from delusions of omnipotence (I do not need you and if I become my only God everyone will idolize me and I myself will not be so cowardly as to have to stoop to ask someone for something), very strong self-centeredness, phases of excessive mania followed by depressive phases and a constant feeling of emptiness.

They are also unfaithful people, serial traitors because their fragile and insecure ego needs constant attention and confirmation.

How can I behave TODAY if I realize that I have or have had a narcissistic / affectively immature parent?

In general, it is difficult to do it alone and therefore a good targeted path is necessary.

PSYCHOLOGICAL THERAPY TARGETED AT
AWARENESS OF THE AFFECTIVE DYNAMICS
IMPLIED IN PATHOLOGICAL NARCISSISM AND
ON THE CONSEQUENCES THAT IT IMPLIES,
FOCUSING ON A PATH OF IDENTIFICATION AND

INDIVIDUAL AUTHORIZATION, BUT ALSO
DIRECTLY TO HEALTH RECOVERY.

Some advice:

Know your "enemy": once we have identified what our parent's basic defects are, we will feel less responsible, less guilty and therefore less manipulable. IT'S NOT MY FAULT. Repeat it often.

Manage Anger: With mindfulness, it is easy to bring up anger and resentment. Revenge and revenge only serves to keep narcissistic dynamics alive, they are of no use to anyone, not even you. These parents also have an emotional problem, "it is not their fault" we say, even if understanding does not mean justifying, but often getting out of it.

Always focus on the emotions you feel, GIVE THEM CREDIBILITY and never the words said or on the facts: this is because in narcissism a process called GASLIGHTING takes place and that is a devaluation and denial of the feelings of the other with the aim of confusing him and therefore managing him or controlling him more easily, often with pitfalls, psychic intrigues or emotional traps.

Set boundaries: by resisting his provocations (STOP PSYCHIC ATTACKS) you will take away the excuse to abuse you emotionally or to control you. This is why you have to let any controversy drop and be clear in your communication, assertive and never argumentative or angry or REACTIVE, because at that point, the dynamic starts. Sometimes it is really necessary to physically distance yourself from him / her, until the dynamic self-extinguishes.

Narcissists are difficult to change, indeed they do not change, but without an audience, their ridiculous mask crumbles, which hides shame, insecurity, fear and low self-esteem, all characteristics that they project onto others.

Often these are people who in turn have been psychologically or physically abused and therefore it is important to develop adequate awareness, a sense of forgiveness, compassion, but also a healthy DETACHMENT, this is because hatred and revenge partly destroy ourselves too, and this makes no sense because the chain of pain would continue.

NARCISSISTIC PARENTS AND AFFECTIVE MANIPULATION

Parents who expect gratitude from their
children (there are even those who demand it)
are like usurers: they willingly risk the capital in
order to collect the interest.

Franz Kafka

We often speak in psychology of "narcissism", of disastrous relationships that are established between two beings that will end up playing a "love play" in the role of victim and executioner. Obviously when we talk about "love relationships" it is also extended to parental relationships, friendship, kinship, etc. and not just to couple's relationships.

For those who are familiar with narcissism and energetic vampirism, it is clear that the two figures often coincide even if they are defined with different names. In fact, the narcissist ends up by psychologically destroying his victim, often unaware that he is not experiencing a love relationship but a nightmare that will soon end up sending her to analysis.

Vampirism, on the other hand, can be seen as the subtraction of forces by an executioner defined as a "vampire" and which causes in the victim states of abulia and total inability to react in the face of the offenses and manipulation that this uses to completely cancel the others will. Whether they are vampires, whether they are narcissists, the result is the same and therefore it becomes important to understand the modalities and characteristics, in order to observe with other eyes what is happening in one's personal sphere through the parental figures.

TYPES OF NARCISSISTIC PARENTS

Narcissistic parents are mainly divided into two categories. Intrusive parents and disinterested ones. Both of these types of narcissistic parents harm their children incredibly.

- **Intrusive parents**: they are those who see no boundaries between themselves and their children. Children are seen as an extension of their parents and not as individuals. For infants and toddlers this is fine - in fact, young children often don't see themselves as separate from their parents. The problem, however, is that this type of narcissistic parent will never take into account the age of the child, will not have problems asking overly personal questions, reading e-mails and personal notes of the child, even when he is grown up.

- **Disinterested parents:** they are those who do not care much for their children. Unlike pushy parents, the disinterested parent sees boundaries between himself and his child and has no interest in him. Often, a disinterested parent does not help their child even with personal cleanliness, does not teach him about hygiene, or does not help him with homework. This type of parenting can be confusing and disorienting for children. A child can grow up with the feeling that he is not loved, that he is not cared for, compromising his approach to future relationships with his insecure relational mode.

Characteristics that identify the narcissistic parent:

1) The narcissistic parent has difficulty empathizing and creating meaningful bonds. Because their needs prevail, they have little room for the needs of others. This makes it nearly impossible for a narcissistic parent to understand emotions and meet the physical and emotional needs of their children.

2) The narcissistic parent attributes the success of his / her child to himself. In the mind of the narcissistic parent, he / she is sacrificing everything for his / her child and the child must reciprocate by acting above expectations. Early advances are seen by the narcissistic parent as their own, "he's an excellent footballer - they're my genes. I was also a sportsman".

3) Narcissistic parents need to be in control. It doesn't matter of what. The narcissistic parent controls his / her child by dictating how he / she should feel, how to move and what

decisions to make. This can lead to an adult child becoming insecure, not knowing what to want or not want in their life. Children of narcissistic parents as adults have great difficulty becoming independent and making their own decisions.

4) Narcissistic parents emotionally blackmail their children. The narcissistic parent is often lenient, condescending, and sweet if (when) their child behaves as the parent wishes. In any case, the moment the child becomes disobedient, the narcissistic parent becomes bitter and harsh. This alternation of "I love you, go away" creates insecurity and dependence in the children of narcissistic parents.

HOW NARCISSISTIC PARENTS BEHAVE WITH THEIR CHILDREN

The typical mechanism that the narcissist exercises over a child is control. There are many ways in which the narcissistic parent controls their child. These control mechanisms include:

Codependent control: "I need you. I cannot live without you". This prevents children of narcissistic parents from having any kind of autonomy and living their own lives.

Control with guilt: "I gave my life for you. I sacrificed everything". This control creates the feeling of obligation / constriction in children. As if they "owe something" to their narcissistic parents and behave in a way that will certainly make them happy.

Control with emotional abstinence: "you are deserving of my affection ONLY BECAUSE you behave as I expect you to." So as long as their children behave correctly, the narcissistic parent will love them. This affection disappears the moment the child does not match expectations.

Control over the result: "we must work together to obtain a result". These results are often the results, dreams and fantasies of the narcissistic parent. The narcissistic parent lives indirectly through the life of his / her child.

Explicit control: "Obey me otherwise I will punish you". The children of narcissistic parents must do what they are told or they risk shame, guilt, anger, or even physical violence.

Emotional incest control: "You are my true love, the only one, the most important person to me." The opposite-sex parent causes the child to fulfil their unmet needs.

Beyond the control mechanisms there are other typical behaviors that the narcissist performs to the detriment of their children:

- Compulsive lying
- Ignore them or annihilate them
- Neglect their needs
- Make them feel unimportant
- Model children to an "ideal" image
- Promote and foster a relationship of dependence between parents and children
- Distort the concept of "love"
- Handle for pleasure
- Say one thing one day and another the next day
- Be unreliable

- Use the child's vulnerability (especially when it is small) to exploit it
- Insult, subtly or not
- Ignore personal needs
- Treat others as objects and not as people
- Make your child feel like he's crazy
- Never grow up

SCENARIOS FOR THE ADULT CHILD OF NARCISSISTIC PARENTS

The children of narcissistic parents have not seen their emotional needs met; they have become 'mini adults'. If the parent has long practiced emotional abuse and if the child has not received adequate support (has not had psychological help or other healthy role models) there are two possible scenarios for the adult child of narcissistic parents.

1) The child grows up with narcissistic traits and becomes a narcissistic parent for their children. The cycle of narcissistic abuse continues.
2) The child becomes a "hidden" or "overturned" narcissist who remains codependent and may seek violent relationships with other narcissists.

It is very important for a grown-up child to recognize that they have had a narcissistic parent and to look within themselves, in order to recognize that they have never learned how to relate correctly to feelings and start interacting with them.

Here are some important tips that children of narcissistic parents can follow:

Learning to love each other: the first step that a child of narcissistic parents must take is to start a process of 'mourning' where they elaborate that they did not have a parent who loved them because they were unable to do so, depending on their pathology. The adult child of a narcissistic parent will therefore have to learn to love that little child inside him as the narcissistic parent never did.

Stop hoping that the narcissistic parent will change: he / she will not change. Insisting on a change from the parent is a behavior that leads nowhere except to waste energy by increasing anger, frustration and discomfort.

Stop being afraid of your parent: the children of narcissistic parents must realize that the fear they feel is an emotion that has been attributed to them by their parents. They have to work to erase this fear, get rid of this feeling that conditions them and start taking their life back in their hands.

Find a psychologist or therapist specialized in the treatment of adult children of narcissistic parents: it is very important to ask for help from professionals specialized in the treatment of children of narcissistic parents who know how to illustrate the typical mechanisms of anger, fear, guilt, anxiety that are the basis of the relationship with a narcissistic parent and help them manage them in the most functional way for their well-being.

Working on guilt: Guilt is the worst enemy of an adult child of narcissistic parents. This may be the hardest to fight of all feelings, but it has to be done. Adult children of narcissistic parents will always have to remember that their needs are important, they will have to learn to be respected and to ask for what they need. They will have to stop feeling guilty about not wanting to stay in touch with their parent (in cases of severe abuse it is the only healthy choice for their mental well-being) or when they set clear boundaries in cases where the narcissistic parent is particularly invasive.

Deciding How to Manage Contact with the Narcissistic Parent: Separating from some sort of codependency that is commonly induced by narcissistic parents can seem difficult. Adult children of a narcissistic parent must learn to choose the type of contact from which is least disabling for their well-being.

Basically, they have two possibilities:

1) total estrangement - no contact with the narcissistic parent (in cases of severe abuse and malaise)
2) measured contacts - contact, but limited interaction with the narcissistic parent

If you choose to have limited contact with the narcissistic parent, it is vital to make sure you follow a few clear criteria:

Create very defined boundaries: children of narcissistic parents should not feel obliged to compensate their parent for having removed them from their life. In these cases, you need to be clear and firm (e.g. with an intrusive narcissistic parent who comes in unannounced, you can tell them you are too busy to meet them). It is also very important not to allow them to rely only on their children as if they were the only ones who can take care of them.

Be careful not to let yourself be influenced by your parents: this means making yourself autonomous in your life choices and learning to carry out your decisions regardless of the approval of the parent without feeling wrong and / or guilty.

Giving information only about what "you need to know": just because your narcissistic parent tells everything doesn't mean it has to be reciprocal.

Protect your children from narcissistic grandparents: If there are children, it is essential to protect them from harmful behavior.

It is very important to point out that each case is different from another. This chapter has provided some general tips. If we find ourselves in this difficult condition and we do not know how to manage the situation it is essential to ask for specialist help from a therapist who can listen to our specific situation and guide us in managing the problem in the most functional way for our well-being.

Bottom line: Being a good mother or a good father. Seeing children for what they are, and certainly not a replica of the father or mother, nor of their broken dreams. We cannot therefore expect them to redeem maternal or paternal ambitions. Children are Souls who have come to this Earth to have their experiences... and not ours. Each of us has had her time, the life of our children does not belong to us.

CHAPTER 2 - FATHER NARCISSIST

If there is a narcissistic father in the house, here's what can happen to the children

In the family with a perverse narcissistic father, only one bright star shines: him. The "black" sun of the family, the partner and children exist only as satellite planets that orbit around him, reflecting his light and grandeur.

Their feelings are never taken into consideration. The children, just like the partner, are "cosified" (a term coined by Marie-France Hirigoyen, family psychotherapist expert in psychological violence), or reduced to objects, "things", to be manipulated and used instrumentally to achieve their own ends and the fulfillment of one's narcissistic needs.

Love, respect, freedom of action and thought are replaced by very serious psychological abuse, sometimes even by physical abuse, by a pressing and perpetual hyper-control and by the continuous subtraction of merits and qualities that are never recognized.

Children, brought into the world to become the extension of the perverted narcissist, can have different functions: to allow the parent to show off his offspring: "look what beautiful children I have generated", or to guarantee him a socially desirable image (marrying and having children then it becomes a requirement only because "the time has come to put my head right" or because "everyone does this").

In some cases, I have been able to see that the family theater is put on because doubts about their own sexuality lead these men to find a woman with whom to procreate in order to guarantee an alleged armor of virility and at the same time an image of "normality" that makes them unsuspected, only to then associate with people of the same sex or transsexuals, outside the home.

In general, outside the home, the perverted narcissist always changes personality and behavior. Suddenly he is able to transform, in a truly disturbing way, into the opposite of what he appears at home. Strangers, in fact, are nothing but an audience to whom to show the best part of themselves, therefore, in front of them he will wear the mask of the attentive, caring, impeccable, smiling father, attentive to the needs of the children and always ready to sacrifice himself for them.

It so happens, at least as long as the children are small, that they are led to act like their parent, to demonstrate to his audience that they have received an impeccable education, as imparted by a being so charming, perfect and brilliant that it cannot be than an excellent father, capable of raising wonderful and above the norm children.

However, while a perverse narcissistic father wants his children to reflect his grandeur, on the other hand he fears confrontation. This happens above all when the children, who have become young adults, reveal their first needs for autonomy and identification, perhaps choosing university or professional paths that he does not approve of, as he feels threatened by them.

Thus, this exemplary father does nothing but crush, through ferocious denigration and devaluation, his own children, so that they do not cloud his grandiose image and so that he can continue undisturbed to be the despotic little king of his family.

Narcissistic fathers, not unlike mothers, love to sow discord among their children, pitting them against each other while they, from the small throne where they sit, watch them destroy themselves, without getting their hands dirty.

Children are constantly competing through constant comparisons. Generally, a "golden child" and a "scapegoat child" are elected.

This golden son obtains the appearance of being loved and, in return, sacrifices himself on the altar of his narcissistic father, believing that he is truly deserving of love and therefore accepting to put his life at his service. Not infrequently, this child is implicitly asked to take on the parent's narcissistic tasks directly, psychologically and / or physically abusing the scapegoat, in order to relieve the narcissistic father from this task.

The scapegoat child, on the other hand, functions as a container of psychic garbage that the narcissistic parent cannot accept. All the parts of himself that the narcissist father cannot accept having are constantly deposited on him: so this child will be incapable, ugly, the less intelligent, brilliant or creative one, too introverted or inadequately extroverted, the boring, inadequate one, awkward, the "unregulated" one of the family.

What unites all children of narcissistic parents, whether they are golden children or scapegoats, is that they are sadly alone. In fact, these children cannot ally themselves with the healthy parent, as the following rule applies in these families:

" If one parent is perverted narcissist, the
other is subjected to it"

The children thus grow up alone, suffer in silence and watch, often helpless, the succubus parent yield to the will of the perverse one. This also happens when the succubus parent possesses qualities that could guarantee an emotionally normal growth of the children, as the satisfaction of the needs of the perverse partner deprives them of the clarity and energy necessary to take care of the children with the emotional attention that is their due.

The perverse narcissistic father succeeds in this intent by manipulating, mystifying, gaslighting or smearing his wife, and continually devaluing her in front of his children. By doing so, he will teach, especially to the male child, that devaluing and minimizing the merits of the mother, sister and then of all the women he will know in his life is normal.

Not infrequently, the narcissism of these fathers harms the sons more than the daughters: this is because the father sees in the child and in the young man an extension of himself, rather than an independent person, with his specificities, dreams, desires, psychic and physical requests to be realized.

In this arid family scenario, what are the possible psychopathological outcomes for children?

Typically, the child of the narcissistic family is animated by a blind rage that can act openly or in a passive-aggressive manner. It is often overcome by overwhelming feelings of emptiness. He feels inadequate and unable. He can also have serious episodes of anxiety and depression or manifest important psychosomatic disorders.

The process of identification with the paternal is always difficult: the father in fact proposes an unacceptable male model and it is not uncommon for the sons of narcissistic fathers to develop problems related to gender identity.

In severe cases, growing up with a narcissistic parent can mean developing the following personality types for children:

Post-traumatic personalities (particularly complex PTSD: this form typically occurs following early, interpersonal trauma such as physical, sexual or psychological abuse, repeated mistreatment, cumulative violence or severe neglect by a caregiver).

Dependent personalities: characterized by pervasive insecurity, low self-esteem, very strong abandonment fears that prevent them from realizing themselves and their individuality.

Counter-dependent personalities: avoidant and detached, disinterested in ties, they deny their own emotional and affective needs, experienced as fragility to be ashamed of.

Borderline personality: characterized by emotional instability, deep mood changes, impulsivity, feelings of abandonment (often associated with an inability to be alone and the extreme need to have a person next to you), rapid idealizations and devaluations of the partner who soon becomes " not present or caring enough", self-injurious behavior, threats and suicide attempts.

Perverse narcissistic parents, as it is easy to imagine, never identify in themselves any kind of responsibility for any psychic disturbances manifested by their children.

Proverbial, in this sense, were the words of the narcissistic father of a patient of mine with a severe border personality disorder who, in the middle of a family therapy session, asserted:

"Doctor, I have been an exemplary father. This one (the daughter, so to speak), is a disaster for our family. With her behavior she throws mud on my family, which is a family of decent people, workers, honest people like my parents and all my ancestors were ".

In short, no introspective capacity, not an ounce of self-criticism in this "exemplary father" (which healthy father would say about himself?) Who went on to give all the responsibility for his daughter's suffering to bad company, to consumer society, to the values of the past that they are no longer there (and God only knows if he would not have accused even the aliens of having kidnapped and corrupted her forever, in order not to recognize that he had generated part of that pain in her)?

Being exposed since childhood to such psychological abuse generates enormous confusion that damages and conditions the emotional life of the children, who remain torn between the desire to disown the abusive father and the sense of guilt "because in any case he is always my father is also he, like everyone else, has a good side".

This is one of the perverse dynamics that leads many daughters of narcissistic fathers to see in perverse narcissistic partners (with whom they often bond once they become adults), that something familiar that makes them, in some way, "feel at home" together with them, preventing them from recognizing and identifying the abuse they suffer.

Healing from intra-family narcissistic abuse cannot be separated from accepting the fact that the narcissistic parent cannot be changed because they simply don't want to. In fact, his own ailment, while imposing the idea of perfection on him, also prevents him from accessing treatment: "If I am perfect why should I need help? - thinks a narcissist - if anything, it's the others who need it! "

Psychotherapy can help the children of narcissistic fathers understand and process what has happened within their family. In the safe and welcoming living room of the therapist one can experience all the pain for the ideal parent that one would have desired and that life has denied, one can recover the relationship with the siblings that the narcissistic parent wanted to make enemies, one can regain trust and make a new alliance with the succubus parent, who is also a victim, and give yourself a new chance to still be a family.

To do this it is necessary to be able to authorize oneself to express anger, sadness and pain that have been repressed or denied for a long time: there are no good emotions and bad emotions, there are only emotions that, if lived to the full and without fear, help us to free ourselves from past and to meet our future. A future in which healthy love is always possible: you just need to give yourself permission to see it and, finally, live it to the fullest.

THE NARCISSISTIC FATHER BEFORE AND AFTER THE DIVORCE

"After the divorce, your son will be reconsidered by the Narcissistic father at least until he begins to grow and distance himself. Be prepared, because when the young man distances himself, the father will adopt reactions towards the son that can cause him extreme pain. There is nothing that knocks out a Narcissist more than being devalued and ignored. "

What happens to children who grew up with a narcissistic father during and after a divorce?

This is an important consideration because after you leave the Narcissist behind and recover from the pain, your child will continue to interact with him.

It is not a comforting picture. The healthy parent, who recognizes the Narcissist and knows what to expect from him, by providing useful advice to the child, will help to lessen the pain that otherwise would affect all family members.

Definition of Narcissist:

THE TERM NARCISSIST ORIGINATES FROM NARCISSUS WHO, IN GREEK MYTHOLOGY, FELL IN LOVE WITH HIS OWN IMAGE REFLECTED IN THE WATER. TODAY, THE TERM IS USED TO DESCRIBE A PERSON CHARACTERIZED BY SELF-CENTEREDNESS, VANITY, PRIDE AND SELFISHNESS.

Signs that your child's father is a narcissistic person:

- has an exaggerated self-esteem.
- has a tendency to exaggerate his talents.
- has an excessive need for admiration from others.
- feels excessive envy of others.
- he constantly believes that he is the object of envy from others.
- has a major lack of empathy.
- is always in a position of right and this also applies to interpersonal relationships.
- appearances matter a lot to him.

The Narcissist's Source of Nutrition:

the Narcissist's nourishment is the people around him; they help him to be the center of attention and reflect the importance he gives to himself. The Narcissist's sources of nourishment are usually family members, spouse, co-workers (especially those with a humble attitude), and friends. The characteristic that all these people have in common is that they idealize, overestimate and believe everything that the narcissist tells them. The moment these people begin to ask questions, doubt or disagree with him, they lose the interest of the narcissist and stop being his source of nourishment. The children of the narcissist are his basic source... they are always there, they have his genes, they respect him without questioning him and... wow! ... they even look a little like him.

The narcissistic father:

Narcissistic fathers see their children as simply an extension of themselves. This situation often includes the parental expectation that their children are just as perfect as they perceive themselves to be. They are not able to see children as individuals with their own ideas, for obvious reasons this becomes highly destructive as the children approach adolescence. Every decision they make is examined by the narcissistic father, every dream, idea or hint of independent thought is dismissed by the father if it does not conform to his ideas.

Narcissistic disapproval:

if the son of a narcissist chooses a course of study that does not meet expectations such as medicine, law or architecture, the father will show his disapproval to everyone. The father may go so far as to pretend that his son does not go to college.

His studies are not perceived as real because they are not what he was told to do. You can imagine where this lead. The son is strongly pressured in the search for any moral or emotional support from the father but he is totally unable to give it. Narcissistic fathers are able to approve only what reflects the image they want to give or what puts them in the spotlight. Certainly, if the son chose jurisprudence for his studies, the narcissist would boast about it because it would have a positive reflection on him.

A daughter's experience with a narcissistic father after divorce:

The daughter of a friend of mine had the "pleasure" of meeting one of her father's longtime friends .... the ensuing conversation was humiliating. The man asked her why she left the university and the reason for so many tattoos. When she explained that she did not leave the university but that she attended evening classes he replied that those courses were not real (worthless). Interestingly, her father had told her exactly the same thing the previous weekend.

This example shows how toxic the narcissist can be and how much it affects those around him, in this case the friend. The conversation left the girl with a feeling of great frustration. The narcissistic father can be extremely charming and funny. As long as children are a source of energy for their narcissism then they will benefit from its charm.

Parent's concern for their children can quickly turn into neglect and abuse. In fact, once they become adults, they will cease to provide energy when they begin to contest the ideas of the parent or simply to have their own, even if this is a normal phase of growth of a child the narcissist will not accept it. The narcissist asks his children to be worshiped.

Divorce and the Narcissistic Father:

During a divorce, the position of the other parent is very difficult. Narcissists will wear themselves out for a long time over custody of children, distort reality, and lie to maintain the devotion of children. After all, the narcissist is insecure, after divorce parenting becomes a very popular competition field: the veneration of children is at stake. Their egos are vulnerable and they lash out at all who reject the perfect image they have of themselves.

If you have filed for divorce, you can bet that their anger will focus on you. Thus, what begins as a kind of possession can escalate to a destructive pattern of parental alienation. It is fair to say that a narcissistic parent is more likely to use parental alienation as a method of retaliation than a regular parent. What begins as constant, possessive attention from the father inevitably becomes rejection as children become adults.

IMPACT ON CHILDREN WITH A NARCISSISTIC FATHER:

When the child is on the verge of becoming an adult and taking flight, there will likely be a conflict between the narcissistic parent and the child.

If the child (now a young adult) is not readily available to satisfy the father's requests, he will be subjected to abuse which can be verbal, emotional, mental and sometimes even physical.

The repercussions on the child will be seen in the form of:

- low self-esteem
- stress
- insecurity
- lack of confidence

If the child is no longer good for the narcissist, then he is no longer good at anything and is told this openly. The narcissist can go further by telling anyone willing to listen to him how disobedient and terrible his son is.

How badly he treated him.

It is common to hear the narcissist define themselves as the victim.

Narcissists may even use other people or sources to "make him think".

This creates a huge source of stress for the child as he is challenged by family and friends who believe the narcissist's tales. But mitigating the terrible words of the narcissistic parent to be able to tell his story leaves the adult child defensive and frustrated. The child's self-esteem and confidence are further eroded.

It is important that you, as a healthy parent, recognize that this treatment is abusive.

Talk to your child about narcissistic abuse:

Explain to the child that he is not responsible for the abuse, that he did nothing wrong, and that he does not deserve this abuse. Remind your child that it is right for him to stand up for himself. Getting him out of the abusive situation is the key to helping him fight back. Provide your child - whatever their age - with the skills and tactics to handle the narcissistic parent. In extreme cases, the adult child may need to distance themselves from their parents in order to maintain a healthy lifestyle and recover.

TIPS FOR YOUNG ADULTS WITH NARCISSISTIC FATHERS

- Anticipate conflict and practice staying calm and keeping explanations simple;
- Learn the personality type of your narcissistic parent and make sure you understand that it is NOT your problem;
- Keep your expectations of the parent low;
- If there is a need to negotiate something with the narcissistic parent, always start by pointing out what the benefits are for him;
- Establish and maintain boundaries to reduce emotional interference and bullying;
- It's okay to say "no" to your father;
- Know when it's time to leave to live healthily;
- Keeping your distance allows you to have a limited but better relationship with the narcissistic parent;

- Try to understand that the narcissist's apology is often an insincere act and that the abusive patterns will probably repeat themselves;
- Narcissists often express love with money;

TIPS FOR HEALTHY PARENTS

- Love your child unconditionally
- Be a source of moral support
- Model normal behavior
- Praise your child's independence and decision-making ability
- Allow him to make mistakes
- Recognize the abuse
- Continue to teach him the "etiquette" of relationships

It is important to understand the destructive behaviors of the narcissistic father and their impact on your children. Especially after divorce, when the narcissist can become even more insecure and abusive.

Knowing that as your children grow up, conflict with the narcissistic father is likely to escalate.

Recognizing that these behaviors are abusive and educating your child on how to best manage the narcissistic father will help them overcome the continuing difficulties this relationship will bring.

THE BEST TACTIC?

CONTINUE TO MODEL NORMAL PARENTAL BEHAVIOR

THE JEALOUSY OF THE NARCISSISTIC PARENT TOWARDS THE CHILDREN

This is a very difficult topic to touch on, because it is difficult to admit (both as a child and as a parent) that a parent can have envy or jealousy towards their children: a matter of possessiveness and excessive love or of poor self-realization and frustration?

The narcissistic mother,

(famously identified metaphorically as RAIN,
SPIDER, OCTOPUS).

This jealousy is not always aware, that is, it can be unconscious and detectable by a whole series of dynamics, which the child of a parent with a narcissistic personality has to face with a certain regularity throughout his life.

Oh yes, because while a partner can leave it, a job can change it, a parent cannot totally exclude it (except in rare cases where it is desirable) and inevitably we must both protect ourselves from its manipulative tendencies and maintain a healthy relationship with them and with us themselves.

The triangulation of the narcissistic mother in the couple

Why do we need to put boundaries with this type of parent?

The underlying feeling is the persecutory one of "feeling trapped", the constant "tension" for something you will say / do or not say / do and that will certainly disappoint him / her in seemingly relaxed situations and / or contexts (dinners, anniversaries , parties ..), but which turn out to be the terrain of ferocious aggressive dynamics, leading you into a paradoxical game in which - for example - you are offered a lunch and then you are accused of lacking effort made to prepare it if you do not gratify your mother or dad as he / she had imagined. It seems that these people with their fluctuating mood, their sudden changes of ideas or attitude, manage to alter the serenity and family calm, but above all the mental serenity of those who live with them.

Description of the Narcissistic Parent

For a narcissist / narcissistic parent being in the center of attention is essential, so when this is not possible, they become anxious and more or less consciously mature negative emotions.

The lack of awareness of their negative emotions often results in incoherent and bizarre acting out behavior, dramatically staged, (sudden illness, presumed lack of respect perceived or suffered by diners or guests ...) that make everyone uncomfortable or covertly devaluing behaviors that they make everyone feel ashamed and, in any case, ruin the day.

For example, if you give a gift to a narcissistic father / mother, instead of appreciating them, they will devalue the positive elements with determination by highlighting - even in an unpolite way - only the negative ones (uhh that's cute! Gloves! I have, I think I have a duplicate, but patience, what matters is the thought!).

Narcissists go out of their way to draw attention to themselves, to create discomfort, tension or to spark an argument, especially if you are happy at the time, no matter if you are celebrating your 18th birthday, your wedding or your funeral, a narcissist will only see a stage on which to perform and if he cannot be the protagonist then he will have to be the villain or the victim, turning you into the villain.

AFFECTIVE BLACKMAIL OF THE NARCISSISTIC PARENT

They have no real interest in your emotions and your happiness unless they are the protagonists or the primary reason, but instead feel the immediate need to give your sentences or intentions negative interpretations to seek a hostile confrontation. In this desperate attempt to raise their deficient self-esteem, they also lose their sense of reality. It is therefore not uncommon for a narcissist to put himself on a par with his son / even if he is 6/7 years old .. so, if a child feels happy to have been at her aunt or cousin's house because she knows how to make cakes, the mother narcissist will not limit herself to empathically sharing her joy, on the contrary she will take the opportunity to ask her daughter if her cakes are good and if so how much more than aunt's? The important thing is competition, comparison, not the happiness of the daughter.

It almost seems that narcissists are terrified of harmony and serenity, so they either have to focus on themselves or they have to spoil it.

In the worst cases, the narcissist will try to make scorched earth around you, because your friends or partners or relatives are potential enemies for them or in general a threat to the competition in the exclusive relationship with you.

IRONIC EXAMPLE OF FATHER NARCISSIST

The constant denigration of the external world is aimed at generating in you fear of novelty and distrust in your neighbor and with it, your condition of psychological or emotional dependence is indirectly strengthened.

Noteworthy is the constant sabotage of your work or creative projects; For example, if you feel joyful because you have bought a camera and decide to devote yourself to the hobby of photography, the narcissist will scold you for the money spent, the uselessness of the project or will judge you idle and childish.

Another important fact is the tendency of narcissists to interfere with the growth of children, especially as regards the formation of the couple, marriage and children.

The narcissist does not want to grow old, it only recognizes itself in the role of a seductive and independent adult, so if you grow up and become independent, they fall into absolute panic. If you try to grow, to combine something in your life, the narcissist will at first show collaborative and enthusiastic and gradually more and more critical and devaluing or even worse manipulative: they know how to do better than you, they have already been there, they put themselves in front of you in every situation and interfere with your role as wife / husband, father / mother with grandchildren.

If you split up, fail at work, something bad happens to you, you can't follow your children all the better. They will still feel protagonists and will always be able to hear us reminding you "what they did for you and for your love" or in the most serious cases "you were stupid in your place I would not have been wrong".

INTERGENERATIONAL TRANSMISSION OF THE NARCISSISTIC DYNAMIC IN THE FAMILY

It is not uncommon for a narcissist to ally against you with your partner or to subtly insert themselves into your couple dynamics with the unconscious goal of regaining the position of dominance over the child; the techniques are varied: from the devaluation of the partner, to triangulation, victimization or the insinuation of doubts about his / her reliability: "he / she is not good for you, he / she does not understand you..." etc... "betrays you".

If your partner is not strong enough or he / she also has narcissistic injuries or insecurities (most likely if you have been a victim of narcissism since childhood), the matter gets worse, because it is much easier for the parent to initiate. quarrels, competitions, triangulations and conflicts.

Conflict is a form of nourishment for narcissists because through comparison and contrast, he feels he is regaining a position of dominance over you and the bad news is that the more he feels inferior to someone, the more he acts in a way to stir up conflicts and stage dramas.

You are confused because narcissists alternate periods of great generosity and momentum with periods of intense sadistic malice and this shows that neither of the two attitudes fully describe them, but it tells you something about the difficulty of integrating these two ambivalent images into your mind.

These parents weigh, tire, usurp, empty, disappoint, confuse, invade, judge, hurt, because basically they procreate only to have someone to idolize and care for them.

We understand that probably these sick parents behave badly but have no really malicious intent (except for rare cases / malignant narcissists) indeed perhaps they are convinced that they are acting for your good and theirs, but the result does not change: you always feel wrong / and, guilty, uneasy, trapped, lacking or anxious.

THE LONELINESS OF THE CHILD VICTIM OF NARCISSISTIC ABUSE

Narcissists are also very difficult to help; they devalue psychiatrists, psychotherapists, they avoid advice; you are always the sick ones, the wrong ones ... so if you are in a situation of this type, worry about yourself, rehabilitate yourself and allow yourself to be happy, but above all, to not to be WRONG, to live and not feel for this constantly guilty.

NARCISSIST AND CHILDREN: A COMPLEX RELATIONSHIP

Self-centered, manipulative, and terribly charming - this is how the narcissist shows himself. It is more than obvious that living with such a person is very difficult. Entering into a relationship with him is exhausting and the situation is further complicated if you have to carry on a family with them.

The narcissist due to his personality characteristics is completely unsuitable to fill the complicated role of parent, since it requires dedication to the other and empathic attention.

A narcissistic father or a narcissistic mother are anaffective parents and therefore risk negatively affecting the development and growth of the child.

Increasingly, however, narcissists are marrying (despite the fact that most of them end up divorcing) and embarking on the adventure of parenting.

How to defend yourself from a narcissist?

A useful first step is to try to understand the behavior patterns adopted by narcissistic parents towards their partner and children, in order to act correctly.

Who is the narcissist really?

If you try to ask acquaintances and friends to describe the narcissistic partner, you will receive an ambivalent picture, which is divided between those who "cheer" him and those who hate him.

In truth, a narcissist never really opens up to anyone, he thinks it is useless and therefore no one will ever know him well enough to be able to make an "objective" judgment on him.

To better understand the characteristics of a narcissist it may be useful to refer to the diagnostic criteria illustrated in DSM V.

This type of pathology, known for its eccentricity and self-centeredness, has another side of the coin, one of weakness and insecurity.

Narcissists, therefore, appear grandiose but are extremely fragile; they exalt themselves but feel tragically alone and experience a strong sense of unease and insecurity which, instead of being verbalized, is hidden from the world by the mask of grandeur that the narcissist loves to wear.

narcissistic parent

On the side of the son

The child of a narcissistic parent must suffer from a lack of sensitivity and empathy and often find themselves having to contend with the attempts of manipulation and control typical of the narcissist.

Control can manifest itself in different shades:

Co-dependent control "I need you. I can't live without you", implicit in what seems like a message of affection, is real blackmail: the child even feels responsible for the existence of the narcissistic parent (reversal of roles) preventing an autonomous and balanced development.

Control aimed at guilt: "I gave my life for you. I sacrificed everything". In this case, more than with blackmail, the narcissistic parent plays on the guilt of the child who is unfairly blamed for being the cause of the parent's (alleged or real) sacrifices. Obviously, these kinds of statements will make the child feel incredibly guilty. He will feel helpless in the face of the guilt that the parent attributes to him. The child is therefore overwhelmed by a weight that he is unable to manage and, in any case, he will always feel indebted to the parental figure.

Control devoid of affection: "you are deserving of my affection just because you behave as I expect you to do." This threat leads the child to believe that he is worthy of affection not as a person and child, but only in relation to his behavior. This is the worst blackmail that a parent can do to a child, as it instills in him the idea that selfless love does not exist and he, internalizing this idea, can only follow in the footsteps of the narcissistic parent.

Control aimed at the result: "we must work together to obtain a result". Also, in this case the message is extremely ambiguous: if on the one hand it seems to be a collaboration, on the other it implies the control of the parent over the child, which occurs with a very strong and authoritative physical, emotional and mental presence.

Explicit control: "Obey me otherwise I will punish you" In this case there is no ambiguity: either you obey or you succumb to the punishments.

Emotionally selfish control: "You are my true love, the only one, the most important person to me." The parent makes the child feel responsible for his happiness, and gives a distorted and sick idea of parental love. Sometimes the child feels compelled to intervene to regulate the happiness of the parent and therefore plays the role of the family adult. This role reversal is once again both unnatural and harmful to the child.

On the partner's side

If everyone knows the characteristics of the narcissist, it is more helpful to understand what is best not to expect from this type of partner. Living with a narcissist is one of the most devastating experiences that can exist.

For what reason?

The narcissist is first and foremost unable to love unconditionally, if you are with a narcissistic partner, he will inevitably make you feel inferior, submissive and in error: those who are with him feel inadequate and terribly at fault.

The narcissist is never a present and caring partner because his mental setting prevents him from feeling true and sincere empathy and therefore, he is unable to tune in to the other's emotions. It is utopian to think that he can open up or that he somehow admits that he was wrong: discussions are his forte, a field where it is better to avoid challenging him. Manipulative and sneaky, he will be able to turn the tables every time you attack him, making you feel guilty and perhaps forcing you to apologize to him.

Unfortunately, the narcissist is unable to contemplate any interest other than his own and knows how to play his cards at the right time: it is entirely plausible that he has seduced you brilliantly and that he has shown his "dark side", living together.

Hardly any narcissist still wants their partner sexually after cohabitation, much less after having a child: what used to be an overwhelming and slightly insane passion can quickly turn into the most boring of routines.

Precisely for this reason, it must be remembered that the narcissist is terribly prone to betrayal: the constant need for confirmation pushes him to always seek new emotions. Occasional relationships, infatuations and online encounters are the most frequent situations, but they are almost always artfully concealed: for him to shatter a reality such as a stable relationship, which gives him security and advantages, is very risky and therefore unlikely.

CO-PARENTING WITH A NARCISSIST

The difficulties of sharing the experience of parenting with someone with narcissistic personality disorder are not minor and the situation can become even more complicated in the event of a divorce.

Becoming aware of the narcissist's dysfunctional tactics can be helpful in protecting the parent trying to juggle this situation.

Once these relationship patterns are identified, it is easier to co-parent with a narcissist. Some tips simply serve to not succumbing, others to counteract its manipulations.

It is necessary to put oneself in the perspective of expecting direct or indirect attacks. More specifically, preparing can help you ignore all forms of manipulation and attack, because the narcissist acts this way solely to provoke you.

If he succeeds, he is able to provoke an overreaction in you that will quickly lead you to the wrong side. The person with narcissistic problems loves to put everyone up against it and the same goes for everything related to the mom-dad-son triad. Often his arguments can be particularly difficult to counter, they are very well argued and are meant to provoke you.

Identify all potentially dangerous situations for your child and his health and intervene, instead overlook trifles so as not to generate unnecessary conflicts.

Don't succumb to threats or guilt. Those with Narcissistic Personality Disorder want to spoil the party while you are enjoying your kids. Ignore his calls.

Establish a clear boundary and protect time spent with your children.

As already highlighted above, the "Narcissus" prevails in almost all discussions and does so naturally, since it is inherent in his style of reasoning to completely exclude empathic feeling: it is impossible for him to try to put himself in someone else's shoes.

Do not forget that you are the empathic parent, it will not always be easy but this quality of yours is important for a balanced growth of your child and must be preserved and preserved, despite everything.

NARCISSISM AND NARCISSISTIC ABUSE: SYMPTOMS, CONSEQUENCES ON THE VICTIM AND TREATMENT

Many of us have heard of narcissism at least once in our lives.

Apparently, it may seem an annoying phenomenon due to the eccentricity that surrounds it but, if you are not careful, you risk falling into abuse. This can become a source of suffering for others, as well as, albeit unconsciously, for the subject in question.

Let's see in detail all the aspects that characterize the "narcissistic abuse syndrome".

What is meant by narcissism?

It is a term that hides in itself a vast number of meanings, based on the use one wants to make of it.

Generally, the term is used to describe a problem that a person experiences in relationships with others, with himself or with his partner.

In the field of everyday life, the term narcissism is often associated with selfishness, vanity and presumption.

When considered within a social group, he often wants to emphasize an elitist or indifferent attitude towards the condition, thought and point of view of others.

In a purely psychological field, there are different stages, both to describe what normal love for oneself should be, and the excessive and completely unhealthy self-centeredness due to a strong perception of oneself.

Who are the narcissists?

These are people with a strong ego and with an excessive need for consideration and a need for admiration.

People with a narcissistic personality structure are represented by 3% of the world population and are mostly male.

Narcissists have the deep conviction that they are superior to others and, therefore, have no care or interest in the feelings of others, regardless of whether they are loved ones like family or strangers.

Narcissists see people as mere objects to use whenever they feel the urge to satisfy their desires for narcissistic grandeur.

Studies on Narcissism

Let us consider the considerations made by the pioneer and father of psychoanalysis, Sigmund Freud.

In his first essay on this phenomenon, "Introduction to Narcissism" published in 1914, Freud speaks of primary and secondary or protracted narcissism. According to the scholar, the first type of narcissism would be an intermediate phase between autoeroticism and all eroticism, that is an emotional and sexual predisposition directed by a subject towards other individuals from whom he is able to derive pleasure and satisfaction, in which the child pushes all his erotic drive on himself before diverting it to others. In this phase, a first sketch in a truly narcissistic sense of the ego begins to appear. The second type of narcissism, on the other hand, concerns adulthood and has as its only term of comparison the turning back of every thought or drive on the ego.

Among the most recent scholars of our days, about the phenomenon of narcissism, we must include H. Kohnut, who in PSICHE "defines the narcissistic state of the mind as a libidinal investment of the self, which has no pathological characteristics but represents an organization which expresses an attempt to deal with those irregular maturational situations that inevitably tend to idealize the parental image ". After this premise, correlated by appropriate studies, let's now turn to the problem of the narcissistic abuse syndrome.

Definition of "Narcissistic Abuse Syndrome"

First of all, what do we mean when we talk about "narcissistic abuse"?

It is defined narcissistic abuse syndrome or TDN (or trauma from narcissistic abuse) or, in the English equivalent, NVS (narcissistic victim syndrome), that particular psychic condition that characterizes a subject who is in a relationship with a so-called "affective manipulator ".

BORDERLINE CHILDHOOD

According to some scholars it would be a disorder similar to post traumatic stress disorder (PTSD).

Specifically, it is a form of thought control that uses a precise language created specifically to emotionally deceive another individual, or the victim, in order to plagiarize his mind for the satisfaction of the desires of those who abuse him.

Scientific definition and symptoms

According to the DSM-IV the Narcissistic Abuse Syndrome is attributable to the category of personality disorders.

According to this diagnostic criterion, those with a narcissistic personality disorder have an absolute pervasive sense of grandeur and a need to feel admired, as characterized by a lack of empathy that usually appears within early adulthood.

This syndrome, according to some, seems to bring with it a sort of induced emotional dependence of a biochemical nature, which in itself is sufficient to determine the symptoms due to an abusive relationship.

Symptoms of Narcissistic Abuse Syndrome

The American psychotherapist Kim Saeed expressed herself on this topic, affirming that some typical characteristics of NAS can be:

- Sadness and despair;
- Hypervigilance, anxiety and agitation;
- Sudden mood swings, irritability, anger, strong sense of shame, self-accusation and guilt;
- Mind in shock, denial and disbelief;
- State of general confusion and difficulty concentrating;
- Sense of isolation and disconnection with the outside world;
- Removal from one's family environment and social group;
- Low functionality that often leads to the loss of work, home and, in the most extreme cases, even children.

Who is involved in this "dangerous game"?

Victim and executioner in Narcissistic Abuse Syndrome

In these cases, there are always two parties: the executioner and the victim.

The narcissistic partner (executioner) seems to manifest a dysfunctional behavior that leads to abuse of his victim in a completely violent, brutal and devoid of any kind of sensitivity. From what has been said it is clear that the second is a weak person, who shows the strong need to feel considered.

Executioner: narcissistic traits

The executioner, who has narcissistic traits, presents:

- a grandiose sense of importance;
- unlimited success fantasies;
- the belief of being special;
- need for excessive admiration;
- the belief that everything is due to him;
- manipulative behavior towards others for their own purposes;
- arrogant behavior or attitudes.

The intent of the abusive narcissists is therefore to take control of the mind of others.

Some authors have speculated that when people have been abused in childhood, they grow up with the expectation that others will sooner or later fulfill all their desires, thinking, in adulthood, that they will finally receive (as if it were their right) what they never had in childhood.

The primary objective of these subjects is in fact to totally dominate the thoughts and any type of need or desire wandering in the minds of others, with the intent of making people act as if they were objects in their possession.

VICTIM: TRAITS AND SYMPTOMS AFTER ABUSE

Victim of the narcissist. What can be defined as the victim of the situation is as if he were then attracted into a sort of spell, a fairy tale in which the subject in question believes he has established a relationship different from the usual, unique, in which to feel considered, understood and also protected. And this does not happen only in relationships of love, but also in those of a working nature, or of friendship.

The person who falls into the trap of an abusive narcissist strongly idealizes the subject he has at his side, as he needs basic security and the abuser does, but unconsciously, to increase his ego, to give nourishment to his brazen need to be admired.

To make the idea better, we report below the thought of one of the victims of this abuse.

"His tender, penetrating gaze lands on me and there is nothing around me anymore. It is a warm, languid, seductive gaze made of implicit promises, of special happiness. Nobody can understand. Nobody knows what I am experiencing and I was lucky enough to meet such a being. And he chose me. Together we are what others will never understand. You are my sun, my moon and the air I breathe. You are in every moment inside of me."

Further reading: Paranoid childhood

" It is the abusive relationship itself that causes the symptoms, not, or not always, only the pre-existing characteristics in the victim, who must never be held accountable", says Dr. Mina Rienzo.

Symptoms experienced by the victim

As psychotherapist Kim Saeed states, among the common symptoms experienced by victims after psychological abuse, we have:

- Anxiety;
- Panic attacks;
- Aggression towards oneself or towards others;
- Food disorders;
- Depression;
- Insomnia;
- Strong sense of guilt;
- Lack of concentration;
- Sense of perennial tiredness;
- Self-esteem equal to zero;
- Obsessive-compulsive attitudes;
- Fear of being alone
- Shame;
- Chronic thoughts related to suicide / homicide;
- Memory loss;
- Cognitive difficulties;
- The horror and the sense of guilt and reluctance at the same time for having loved a monster.

How abusive narcissists do it

But, concretely, how do these executioners manage to establish such dynamics? There are various ways in which they sneakily insinuate themselves into the minds of their victims. Between these:

- By questioning their sanity;
- Removing her from their loved ones, especially the family;
- Making her feel the abandoned partner, to turn out to be their only protectors;
- Discrediting her;
- Doubting their cognitive ability;
- Deeming her incapable of making decisions;
- Neutralizing her desires and needs so that everything is dedicated only and exclusively to them;
- Making sure the victim always finds justification for their narcissistic behavior;
- Totally changing the facts;
- By making the victim have their own happiness as their sole goal.

Evolution of the relationship

The victim initially appears to be an essential resource for his executioner: he becomes the main source of approval.

But this illusion doesn't last very long!

It is a bit like in Cinderella's tale: at the stroke of midnight the carriage turns back into a pumpkin, the horses into mice and the princess into a humble maid. And here, suddenly, like in a summer storm, the perfect relationship becomes a real hell!

The victim of the narcissistic person becomes the preferred target of his executioner and his negative judgment: he is devalued, not considered, denigrated, communication becomes confused or almost absent, which leaves the victim completely destabilized; indifference hurts, isolation becomes a closure in oneself, verbal and, in some cases, even physical aggression is the crowning of the work.

Narcissistic abuse comes to present itself as a real violation, a profanity of that natural naivety of the psychic condition of the subject who suffers and of which he does not realize, which assumes within the couple those connotations of naivety and innocence on which the narcissist can play easily.

Consequences for the victim of narcissism

All this brings with its consequences that are devastating to say the least for the subject who suffers these types of abuse, in terms of self-esteem, affecting and manipulating his thinking ability and penetrating like a worm into the deepest depths of his mind:

"Today again he did not look me in the face, on the contrary he gave attention to another. Why? We were talking, but he was laughing at me with someone else... I felt like I was dying. When he looked at me, I was ashamed. What did I say that was stupid? Fool, maybe I have to learn to shut up. Yes, I will do that, next time I will not ask for anything and I will do it alone. Damn, how long is it until next time? What if he doesn't come? Last time he warned me of the length of his absence. But yes... the next one will be better".

These are just some of the obsessive and recurring thoughts that torment the victim, related to rashes, panic attacks and other symptoms.

INVISIOLE WOUNDS: 6 SELF-DESTRUCTIVE OEHAVIORS IN CHILDREN OF NARCISSISTIC PARENTS

Traumatic childhood attachment experiences (narcissistic, psychopathic, abusive, persecuting or abusive parents) mark people's lives in a definitive way and although the trauma we commonly know is that given by a dominant "traumatic event" (PTSD), we must not underestimate the traumatizing power of relationships.

"Cumulative" traumas (abusive or mistreating relationship experiences repeated over time) have the same effect on the brain as a major traumatic event, such as a bereavement, an earthquake or a war experience.

When it comes to trauma, one immediately thinks of war traumas and post-traumatic stress disorder, but never of the consequences that children who are orphaned by war or who suffer abuse and mistreatment in the family face, in terms of adaptation and survival.

"Trauma is the result of an event or a series of events ("cumulative trauma") or a relational atmosphere ("traumatic atmosphere") overwhelming and difficult to absorb, which renders the subject temporarily powerless and interrupts ordinary operations of coping and defense ".

Carelessness, dysuria, neglect, psychological, emotional or physical abuse are typical behaviors in the narcissistic parent, which generate emotional trauma in the children's brain, which can permanently compromise (based on the severity and recurrence abuse) the functioning of the areas connected with emotional regulation and hyper-vigilance systems (attack-flight).

In adulthood, these children will be attracted to the same patterns of abuse and conflict, simply because the brain "recognizes" the traumatic mnemonic trace and compulsively pushes them to "resolve" traumatic relationship experiences connected in childhood with the abusive parent.

It is sad, but it is as if even today we are looking for love from that parent who never gave it to us, in the hope of saying "then it's not my fault", I deserve your love.

The consequences of abuse on childhood therefore, albeit relational or psychological, are highly harmful and immutable on the emotional regulation systems, on the ability to put boundaries with the outside world and on self-esteem.

Van der Kolk, leading expert on trauma, says that psychological violence impairs the development of cognitive functions of learning, memory, emotional regulation, impulse control and increases the risk in adulthood of developing personality pathologies characterized by intense drama, impulsiveness, propensity to addiction (toxic substances or relationships / emotional dependence) and poor impulse control.

Relational trauma affects above all the functioning of the limbic system (amygdala) and memory (hippocampus) and this is why children who are victims of narcissistic abuse by their parents become humoral, anxious, hypervigilant, hyperactive and dysregulated adults both at a behavioral level, and on an emotional level.

It is as if the brain continues to search for signs of danger in the surrounding environment and in the behavior of the people with whom we relate (paranoid obsessiveness towards the partner or the outside world) without being able to trace the origin of the narcissistic wound or integrate it into the present.

Trauma also has negative effects on the prefrontal cortex which modulates our ability to judge and evaluate reality.

The good news is that the brain is plastic: if today we can consistently benefit from an affective experience and positive relationship (even in the therapeutic relationship that aims at integration and emotional awareness), tenacity causes the brain to adapt synaptic responses to the present, remodeling its circuits and generating new patterns.

Here are some signs that we can consider "alarm bells" regarding our state of psycho-affective well-being and which are almost certainly the result of traumatic relationship experiences with narcissistic parents or in general toxic and disturbing personalities.

COACTION TO REPEAT TRAUMA

Your relationship life seems like a repetition of the patterns you lived in childhood with your parents, even though you promised yourself to be a different person.

The person you initially consider "different" often presents themselves as the "savior", and since your inner child is still looking for their idealized parent ("I'll show you that I deserve your love"), they will be inclined without rationally evaluating the risks to rely on anyone who makes him / her feel safe or desired.

Why does it happen?

On an emotional level, the traumatized inner child seeks an "energetic love bombing" from the other and as an adult tends to consider "normal" and balanced people, as static and boring; is looking for a relationship that gives him the feeling of remodeling all those neurotransmitters of the limbic system, compromised with abuse in childhood and to relive that up & down typical of toxic relationships (I try to idealize you, then I devalue you, I walk away and punish you).

The circuits of serotonin, cortisol, oxytocin, dopamine and adrenaline are chronically compromised.

CHAOS AND ABSENCE OF BORDERS

The abuse experienced in childhood, which tends to recur over time, progressively deteriorates your ability to put boundaries or rather "trains" your brain to withstand psychic, emotional and physical pain, which is why the assessment systems realities of a traumatized adult are compromised.

Example: A slap can happen and the punishment is fair if "I behaved badly", I deserved it and so on.

And why do we develop addiction and especially ON WHAT?

In neuro-scientific terms we depend on the ambivalence of the reward from the outside world, or rather on the fact that abusive partners today re-enact those patterns of idealization, devaluation and abandonment that our parents used to act; for this reason the addiction is established at the exact moment in which the partner's judgment towards us passes from idealizing and positive to "critical and angry"; so then we obsessively try to reposition the thermometer hand on "I'm ok for you, please see how good I am, beautiful? .. see how much I deserve love"?

The problem is that we continue to bleed on the people who caused us these wounds instead of growing.

The abuser's goal in fact - is to keep the game active, not win it, keep the sadistic position of deciding how you will feel today, use you as a joystick of his moods and above all, as a garbage can.

The feeling is the same... "you are here, you are a burden to me.... I have already endured you for a long time, since you need me to exist and I gratify you even just by allowing you in my presence".

It is actually all a bluff. You do not need anyone to live today, not even your parents, both the ghostly ones and those you recreate in order not to face the pain and abandonment, but above all the shame of having felt undeserving of love.

INABILITY TO UNDERSTAND THE DIFFERENCE BETWEEN A HEALTHY LOVE AND A PATHOLOGICAL LOVE.

The search for reward and gratification (praise approval) puts the traumatized child into addiction to love bombing by abusive partners, since everything that child has learned about love is wrong: betrayal, triangulation, punishment, assaults, affective and emotional blackmail etc.

In reality, love is unconditional, free, and you do not have to conquer it continuously by masochistically inserting yourself in relationships in which the abuser becomes the one who acts as a thermometer to your emotional stability.

The point is that you are an emotional addict and for this you still need an evil master or an evil witch who determines the condition of a victim in you, since that condition is the only one you recognize as love. (Relational masochism).

PERFECTIONISM, SELF-SABOTAGE AND EXTREME SELF-CRITICISM

Narcissistic parents are often authoritarian and verbally abusive with the intent to subdue their children and persuade them to do things (or take their side), based on punishment, emotional blackmail or manipulation.

As an adult, therefore, this child will adopt behaviors aimed at seeking the approval of others for fear of being abandoned or considered inadequate, ungrateful towards the partner.

If you are too critical with yourself, if you always justify the behavior of the other by questioning only you, if you give up your joys, goals, pleasant activities for the other or you feel guilty if you are happy, if someone compliments you because you may seem vain, selfish ... well then, your self-esteem has almost certainly been damaged by an abusive relationship in childhood, by a parent who convinced you that someone else's life and survival (children aside) is more important than yours.

These coping strategies (coping with reality) are highly dysfunctional, because they put the child of yesterday back in the position of being abused again today.

INCLINED TO ADDICTIONS

The trauma alters the functioning of the reward systems (reward) for this reason, the traumatized adult is prone to addictions to substances that activate him (exciters) or calm him (sedatives / opiates), since the regulatory systems (especially those of the ANS vagus nerve) are compromised, therefore it is as if today you had to make up for the deficiencies of your nervous system by becoming "the DJ of your moods", but in doing this, you clearly risk being trapped by addiction to dangerous substances or deviant behaviors such as addiction to pathological gambling, online shopping, sex, food etc. (new dependencies).

FRAGMENTATION OF THE PERSONALITY

Those who survive a trauma can develop in adulthood, a series of "sub-personalities", which are the result of the fragmentation of the self, following the abuse to defend that part of the inner child that still feels fragile or to sabotage himself, with the aim of colluding with the will of the narcissistic parent, example: "you are an ungrateful and idle child, you are a misfortune, only I can bear you"; this child, when he grows up, could show traits of shyness and fear of the outside world in order not to refute the parent's thesis, without putting himself to the test and therefore on the one hand without risking to confirm that his mother was right, but not even allowing himself to think at all that may not have. (Internal saboteur).

If you have been the victim of a narcissistic parent or a toxic family system, don't be discouraged! Today you can learn to set boundaries, you can practice low contact (in extreme cases no contact) and recover many parts of you, planning and working on your life with autonomy and patience.

That love, that recognition you were looking for, stop looking for it outside and start looking for it in YOURSELF!!

CHAPTER 3 - SOLUTIONS

10 GASLIGHTING TECHNIQUES TO LEARN TO RECOGNIZE AND DEFEND ONESELF

What is gaslighting?

Gaslighting is a technique by which a person or a group of people try to have more power. To do this, you choose a victim and try to manipulate him, so much so that he doubts his reality. It works much better than you might think. It is a very common technique among manipulators and perverse narcissists, in short, among all those who want to create a cult of their person. To protect yourself, it is important to know their tactics.

Gaslighting is slow, so the victim doesn't realize they are being brainwashed. For example, in the movie Gaslight (hence the term), a man manipulates his wife so much that she thinks she has lost her mind. People who use this mind manipulation technique willfully distort information to assert themselves or to question the victim's mental health, memory or perception of reality.

The manipulative techniques of Gaslighting

Gaslighting is precisely a manipulation technique that tries to undermine the self-esteem and sanity of the other in a subtle way to be able to control and subdue him.

It is useful to know these techniques to be able to identify them and above all to protect yourself from them. Here are the processes used by those who use this type of manipulation.

1) They tell lies without any kind of shame

Someone tells you, for example, a lie. You know full well that this is a lie. This lie is communicated to you with a very serious air. Why is it so obvious? This is the first step; it is the basis of gaslighting. Once you've been told a huge lie, you can't be sure of anything, especially if you are later told the truth. The target? Destabilize and disturb.

2) They deny they said anything, even if you have proof

You know they told you something and you are sure you heard it. But when you remind them of what they said, they deny it again and again, endlessly. This leads you to question the facts and to doubt yourself: maybe it's true that they never said that? The more they do it, the more you doubt yourself, your reality, thus starting to accept theirs.

3) They use what is near and dear to you as a means to reach you

They know how important your children are and how important your identity is to you, and that's where they will start attacking you

4) They wear you out

This is one of the most insidious aspects of gaslighting: it is done gradually, over time. A lie here, a lie there, a sharp comment every time ... And the manipulations start creating doubts in you. Even the smartest and most aware people can be trapped in gaslighting.

It is the principle of the boiled frog of the American philosopher Noam Chomsky, used to describe those who end up passively accepting harassment without realizing it.

5) Their actions don't follow their words

When dealing with a person who practices gaslighting, it is better to take into account their actions rather than their words. Their words have no meaning, they are just words. The problem is, in fact, in their actions (what they do or don't do).

6) They offer you positive reinforcements to manipulate you

The person who manipulates you yesterday told you that you are useless, but today he congratulates you on something you have done. This adds a sense of unease because you will think: "well, finally things are not that bad!" It is a subtle and thought-out technique to destabilize you and, once again, make you question your reality. Be careful what you are praised for - this is probably something that serves the purpose of the gaslighter.

7) They know that confusion weakens people

Gaslighters know that everyone loves to feel stable and balanced. Their goal is to destroy your balance and make you doubt constantly. They know that the most natural human tendency is to turn to the person who makes one feel balanced and stable: the gaslighter also takes advantage of this.

8) They try to turn other people against you

Gaslighters are masters of the art of manipulating people and using those around you to turn them against you. They will make comments like "this person knows you are wrong", or "this person thinks you are useless". Keep in mind that this doesn't mean these people actually said these things - a gaslighter is constantly lying. Use this technique so that you don't know who to turn to or who to believe. They know it well: isolating yourself from others gives them more power.

9) He will tell others that you are losing your mind

Here is one of the most effective tactics of the gaslighter: the latter knows very well that, if he tells everyone that you have lost your mind, others will probably not believe you when you try to justify yourself by evoking his personality.

10) He will tell you that everyone is lying

Telling you that everyone is lying (your family, your friends, the media) will make you question your reality and the people around you once again. You have never met someone capable of such boldness and confidence. So, he's most likely telling the truth, right? No, it is a manipulative technique that causes people to turn to the gaslighter to get the "right" information.

Is the gaslighter aware of his behavior?

It depends on the people. One might think that the gaslighter is not aware of his behavior at all, but this is not always the case. Do you know Dale Carnegie's book, How to Influence People and Make Friends? It provides the foundation for gaining the trust of others, for building new relationships, for increasing your popularity, for getting others to think like you, for increasing your persuasive power, welcoming and making your social relationships pleasant. There is a difference between a pathological manipulative and most of those who have read Dale Carnegie.

That is why it is important to know the techniques used by gaslighters: to better protect themselves. Because even if someone does not knowingly do it, they can still reap the benefits when their victim becomes dependent on him. He feels extremely good when no one holds him responsible for his behavior.

Remember: the fact that a gaslighter is not aware of their manipulative behavior does not make their actions acceptable.

Who is the gaslighter

The gaslighter is identified as a manipulator, he can be narcissistic, passive aggressive or violent, but in all cases, he is a pathological manipulator who could assume such behaviors from an early age and who therefore has a great experience in this sense.

He presents himself as a calculating and very intuitive person, able to read in advance the moves of his victims and therefore able to provide positive or negative messages when necessary, depending on his strategy.

In fact, the goal of the gaslighter is not to annihilate their victims, but to bend them to their will and create a relationship based on dependence, making them better people from his point of view. Feeling therefore superior, he will not accept any criticism towards himself, and if he feels challenged, he will defend his choices as externally imposed necessities.

The gaslighter is a person able to ignite the seed of doubt in the other while at the same time favoring a series of conditions that cause this doubt to increase, leaving the victim at the mercy of confusion and dependence on his executioner.

Another characteristic features the gaslighter has is that of constantly wearing a mask and of being himself a victim of his own manipulations and machinations: in this sense the manipulator lives in a state of perennial acting in which he never reveals the true self, which normally was battered by deep problems in childhood, and which lead him to hope for the possibility of a better and different future in which he can finally get rid of this shell.

In any case, the gaslighter is a person who is unable, precisely because of this sort of alienation from himself, to feel empathy or interest in others or face serious self-analysis: therefore, he cannot be saved by anyone, if not from himself and from therapy to help him.

An example of gaslighting can be that which occurs between an authoritarian or overprotective parent and his child: in this case the parent, who assumes the role of gaslighter, treats the child in such a way as not to allow him to develop his personality. And it can do it using different techniques, first of all the sense of protection, the sense of guilt and the lack of responsibility.

In these cases, parents keep their children in a sort of limbo in which they have no responsibility whatsoever and live as subordinate to their parent, with a bond that is based on ownership, for the parent, fear and guilt, for the child, more than on love and education. Among other things, we have already explored in other chapters how hyperprotective or authoritarian parents can generate other forms of pathologies such as perverse narcissism or passive aggression.

Obviously, gaslighting is also present in other types of relationships such as love and friendships and generates the same dynamics of dependence between a superior and a subordinate.

Also, in this case the relationship is based on fear and dependence and not on a form of affection.

HOW TO RECOGNIZE A GASLIGHTER

We have already explored the main gaslighter manipulation techniques, but here we leave you just a small summary of 3 alarm bells that are easily recognizable even at the beginning of a relationship:

Constant use of little lies. Even small lies carry weight because they indicate that a person does not hesitate to use this behavior even when it is not necessary. Lies are one of the first signs of a toxic relationship and are easily identifiable, but you tend to overlook them. If you are starting a relationship or are in a relationship with a pathological liar the advice is always to ask for help and try to get out of it.

To deny the evidence. The manipulator will tend to always deny the evidence, even when his victim has been the victim of the episode in question or to change the version of events, to instill the seed of doubt in the other.

Pathological jealousy: the manipulator is normally a very jealous person, who prevents the other from living his life, but who, as regards himself, allows himself all the freedoms of the case.

STAGES OF GASLIGHTING

For the manipulation to be truly functional the gaslighter will lead its victim through 3 phases:

Distortion of communication. In the first phase, communication goes through a distortion phase that tries to confuse the victim by alternating positive and negative moments. For example, in the case of a love relationship, the manipulator will present himself as charming and in love, creating fantastic situations, but occasionally inserting destabilizing dialogues or hostile silences, which aim to disorient the victim or at least to insinuate a feeling of involuntary misunderstanding.

The defence. The victim is still lucid enough and not submissive to understand that something is wrong, trying to confront the manipulator with dialogue or other forms of communication, or even walking away. But somehow the confusion instilled by the manipulator is such that the victim will feel able to change his executioner, taking this task as a mission, which obviously is doomed to fail and plunge the victim into the manipulator's trap.

Depression. It represents the last stage of manipulation and normally corresponds to the moment in which the manipulator has complete control over the victim, who believes that indeed everything the abuser says about him is true and therefore yields to the will of the other.

At this point the manipulation reaches its peak and the psychological and / or physical violence becomes chronic and on the agenda: the victim also blindly believes in his abuser and very often sees him as a savior.

EXAMPLES OF GASLIGHTING

Some examples of clinical gaslighting and popular references of studies pertain to some psychological studies including:

According to a study by Marta Stout, gaslighting is frequently used by sociopaths because they have different characteristics, such as the fact that they normally transgress laws and social conventions, they have little empathy and can even be clever liars in hiding their misdeeds. Therefore, they possess those characteristics that make them skilled manipulators.

According to a 1998 study by Jacobson and Gottman, gaslighting is also used by abusive husbands who use it with their wives to deny forms of violence and abuse.

Gaslighting is also used in some cases of adultery according to psychologists Gass and Nichols where husbands using this technique can lead to the emotional breakdown of the wives, in some cases up to suicide.

Another example of Gaslighting was carried out by the Manson family in the United States in the late sixties during their crimes: for example, they entered the homes of residents without stealing anything, but moving the furniture and leaving traces of their passage to sow anxiety.

These are some of the most popular clinical examples of gaslighting that further demonstrate just how destructive and evil this manipulative technique can be.

The consequences and how to recognize that you are a victim

The consequences of gaslighting can be severe. Let's see what are the feelings that can help us recognize that we are a victim of this abuse:

Confusional state: as we have already mentioned, one of the first indications of being a victim of gaslighting is that of feeling confused and doubtful, lost in the inability to realize what is happening.

Feeling worthless: The victim will feel worthless, undeserving of love, and completely dependent on the other.

Tiredness: the manipulations of the gaslighter will make the victim devoid of strength and motivation both physically and mentally.

Shame: the victim's self-esteem is constantly humiliated and having lost the certainty of his emotions, ideas and reality, he will feel constant shame at the very thought of being with other people and will withdraw into isolation.

Dependence and idealization: as previously mentioned, a total dependence between the superior and the subordinate is created between the victim and the manipulator, so much so that the victim tends to idealize his executioner as a savior.

Furthermore, the long-term effects of gaslighting can generate anxiety, depression, isolation and psychological trauma

Gaslighting Examples and How to Defend Yourself

Is there a self-test for gaslighting?

It is difficult to say if there is a self-test for gaslighting, although according to Dr. Ramani Durvasala, just feeling the need to record the conversations or events that happen to us to be sure that we have not made it all up is a clear symptom of be a victim and therefore can be used as a test.

Another clue might be to ask yourself if you recognize some of these phrases and if they have been repeated to you often:

- "Don't be so touchy!"
- "Look, it never happened, you remember wrong!"
- "Look, things did not go this way, but this way."
- "Are you sure you're okay? Why are you saying such strange things?"

Obviously, these are just some indications, the main advice is always to ask for help both from people close to you and from a therapist in case you feel you are victims of any kind of abuse.

How to defend yourself?

How is it possible to defend against a gaslighter?

The first tip here too is always to ask for help from people close to you or a professional in the sector. In addition to this, however, since this type of psychological violence tends to destroy the perception of our reality, we could think of collecting evidence to feel more secure:

- keep a diary in a safe and hidden place to record events
- Record conversations and events with your mobile phone or other voice memo device.
- Take pictures

Email: Emailing the evidence to a trusted person and then deleting the traces may be a good advice not to keep the evidence collected at home.

To defend oneself and rebuild one's identity can take a long time after being a victim of gaslighting but some points of the reconstruction, once out of the manipulator's trap, could be:

- remember that you are never, ever responsible for the abusive behavior of the gaslighter.
- Avoid fomenting discussions about what is true or right with the manipulative person. Learn again to listen to your thoughts and feelings.
- Request the support of a therapist to create together a path of recovery from trauma
- Rebuild relationships with family and friends.

Gaslighting and psychological violence: is it a crime?

Gaslighting and psychological violence are not identified as crimes per se, but are linked to other forms of crime such as family abuse, private violence, threats and stalking and it is therefore important to report them, especially for help. In these cases, it is also important to collect the evidence we mentioned in the previous paragraph in order to be able to provide all the documentation possible.

WAYS TO BUILD RESILIENCE IN CHILDREN WHEN SHARING PARENTING WITH A NARCISSISTIC EX

The tensions of co-parenting with a narcissist

Anyone who has been in a relationship with a narcissist and, through their strength and determination, has decided to end that relationship, feels a deep sense of relief once the trauma is over. Getting away from the pain and negativity that the narcissist brings into their world implies a radical change of life, marking a new reality for these people, capable of overcoming the problems and the anguish experienced.

If you recognize yourself in this circumstance, I know that you live in a state of tangible tension. The impact of such a condition cannot be understated. Co-parenting presents a number of challenges for anyone, and the added difficulty of sharing parenting with a narcissist greatly exacerbates the sensitivity of relationships.

If your relationship recently ended and your partner was an abusive narcissist, it's natural to want to distance yourself as quickly as possible. You've probably endured tremendous pain at her hands and your ex's manipulative and selfish behaviors are almost certain to continue after the breakup.

First, children have the right to know and maintain relationships with both parents. It is important for their identity and their sense of self. If all contact were to cease and your partner went to court, the judiciary would most likely force you to maintain some form of contact to preserve the narcissist's relationship with their children.

Only in very serious circumstances is contact completely forbidden.

To make the situation even more complex, when we decide to cut off all contact between the narcissistic parent and our children, the end result could be counterproductive: children can construct an unduly positive picture of the perpetrator in their fantasies. The risk is that they end up putting this parent on the pedestal, as they are not aware of or have forgotten the negative aspects of narcissistic behavior.

Children may find themselves thinking "the grass is much greener" with the other parent, especially when the one they reside with has been fully charged with all the grueling responsibilities of being a single parent around the clock.

WAYS TO BUILD RESILIENCE IN CHILDREN WHEN SHARING PARENTING WITH A FORMER NARCISSIST

The remainder of this chapter is intended to help out those who share parenting with a narcissist by offering resilience-building strategies and encouragement in children as a way to protect them from the ex's potentially harmful behavior.

The question is, then how do you balance co-parenting with such a person and at the same time instill confidence in your children? Much of the answer lies in knowing how to build resilience within the children themselves.

Resilience is about being able to quickly recover from difficulties and knowing how to deal with setbacks and blocks. In children, resilience begins to develop from an early age. A healthy parent is perfectly capable of helping their children develop it in various ways.

BECOMING THEIR SAFE PORT

First, you need to become a "safe haven" for children, "a place" they can always return to as they explore and learn about the world. Part of being this secure base is allowing our children to navigate the world - in this case, seeing the narcissistic parent - knowing that they can return to the calm, safe and secure place they started from. This is no easy feat, as it requires us to momentarily put aside our emotions and judgments as we listen to our children's stories of everything that happened while they were with the other parent.

PROMOTING A STRONG SENSE OF SELF, THROUGH:

THE STRENGTHENING OF IDENTITY

An important part of resilience is the child's self-esteem, sense of self and identity. It is essential to allow our children to have a level of autonomy in their lives, giving them the opportunity to demonstrate their responsibility.

THE DEVELOPMENT OF AN INTERNAL COMPASS

Encouraging the mastery of new skills increases self-awareness and self-confidence. This involves developing an internal control compass that the child relies on to understand that he can influence external events instead of being overwhelmed by them - as is often the case with children of narcissistic parents.

THE TEACHING OF THE SKILL OF DISCERNMENT

Developing the ability to discern makes them reject negative messages about themselves, increasing their resilience and more: it provides basic skills on how to manage their relationship with the narcissistic parent.

THE INCENTIVE TO CULTIVATE DREAMS

It is also important that children develop a purpose in life and hope for their future. This aspect can be favored through the definition of objectives to be achieved and the encouragement to dream, to have aspirations.

THE BUILDING OF HEALTHY RELATIONSHIPS

Finally, it is vital that children have access to other healthy relationships outside of their parents. This could be an aunt or uncle, a school teacher, or a spiritual counselor. Building strong, supportive social networks and cultivating healthy and respectful relationships help children understand and set their boundaries. Then they also learn what to expect when they begin to relate to others, including parents.

THE IMPORTANCE OF RESILIENCE IN CO-PARENTING WITH A NARCISSIST

Building resilience in your children instills more strength in the relationship with the narcissistic parent. A resilient person values their self-esteem and makes themselves less vulnerable to manipulation.

As they grow, resilience will help them fight respectfully for the integrity of their self, teaching them to protect themselves from entering into potentially dysfunctional relationships.

Ultimately, it's about giving our children the life skills they will need to set healthy boundaries with the narcissistic parent into adulthood, when they may decide to have a family of their own.

Note: There are evidently some situations where the child's safety is at risk if left alone with an abusive parent and where the risk of serious abuse is too high. In these situations, it is imperative that the healthy parent seeks appropriate legal and professional support to protect the child. It is possible to legally obtain supervised visits, restraining orders or absolute bans from attending between the abusive parent and the child.

LEARNING TO LIVE BEYOND OUR NARCISSISTIC PARENTS

Raising a child of one or more narcissistic parents can make adult life uncomfortable. Hundreds of thousands of us around the world have been the unintended victims of caretakers who only see themselves, and it has devastated not only our mental well-being but also our self-esteem.

Understanding the Narcissistic Parent.

Narcissists are generally grandiose people who lack empathy for those around them, while harboring arrogant, self-centered, demanding or manipulative tendencies. The narcissistic parent is someone who takes it one step further, projecting their insecurities onto their children in a way that marginalizes them or makes them feel inferior or insecure.

Although each case is different, narcissistic parents generally do it in two ways. They may engage in petty or humiliating competition with their children, or they may push their children into mythical competition, pitting them against unmovable standards or constant confrontation that undermines their self-esteem.

However, they achieve their goals, they destroy the way we define ourselves and hinder our ability to create lasting and meaningful connections. However, it doesn't stop there. Toxicity from a self-obsessed parent can follow us long after childhood ends, making it difficult to thrive in a world filled with other broken and unhealthy people. If we are truly seeking to create an environment of happiness and peace, we must learn to overcome their darkness ... but this is a path that requires courage and commitment.

How narcissism manifests itself in our parents.

Live indirectly

Projected superficiality

Narcissists, by definition, are grandiose and this can often mean projecting a superior, superficial image of themselves to the world. They may flaunt themselves in public, pat themselves on the back for their "superior" beliefs or dispositions, or they may flaunt their appearance and material possessions. These people go to great lengths to get ego-boosting attention, even if it comes at the expense of their children and their ego.

Heavy handling

Traditional abandonment

Often, the narcissistic parent may appear to be dominant or overbearing, but some narcissistic parents choose a different path; making sure they are so self-centered that they neglect their parenting responsibilities altogether. This can manifest itself in the form of a career obsession, personal indulgence, or social glitz. However, it happens, the child is left aside and the parent is alone, as they prefer.

Marginalization

They could nitpick, judge, criticize, compare and invalidate their successes or emotions. The common theme is always "you are not good enough and you never will be".

Being too rigid

Zero empathy

Addiction

Some narcissistic parents keep themselves on the edge by expecting their children to take care of them and take care of them for the rest of their lives. These parents can also foster both physical and emotional addiction and could do so through financial or material means. While it is a noble thing to take care of one's parents, the narcissistic guardian achieves this goal through manipulation rather than willful sacrifice, completely ignoring the individual needs of their child.

Jealousy or possessiveness

Chronic self-loathing

Children crave love, but that love hardly comes when it comes to the self-obsessed parent. Unable to satisfy their innate need for affection, these children often seek absolution by sacrificing their self-esteem on the altar of parental narcissism. These become internalized beliefs and thoughts of self-loathing like, "If I were a little quieter, she'd love me more", or "If I fix myself, maybe she'll finally love me ..."

POST-TRAUMATIC STRESS DISORDER (PTSD)

Reflex narcissism

It should come as no surprise that narcissists breed other narcissists. Our custodians are our role models and the first indicators of the type of person we should model ourselves on.

Inability to meet needs

As narcissists make their needs the only important thing in the environment, their children become terrified of themselves and this leads to panic of need. Panic of need occurs when a need is identified and then compulsively buried deep, to be avoided. Then inevitably comes a crisis and the need arises, causing untold problems and the need for constant reassurance.

Insecure attachment

When we are neglected, mistreated, or otherwise removed from our parents' emotions and affections. Likewise, we may also be chasing love, in a complex combination of unpredictability that causes immeasurable damage in our personal and professional lives.

Tendency to please

Those who grow up victims of narcissistic parents often become obsessed with maintaining the happiness of those around them, and this often comes at the expense of their own needs. Some even grow up hating their own needs, believing themselves unworthy or "burden".

Try to disappear

Unlike more aggressive children, extremely sensitive or empathic children respond to self-obsessed caregivers by shrinking and occupying as little space in the world of abusers as possible.

Harmful self-sufficiency

The child who has learned that the parent does not love them is a child who learns that he is the only person in the world he can depend on. When our parents are absorbed in their worlds, we become adults who believe that nobody can be trusted.

The best ways to overcome our narcissistic parents.

Growing up as a victim of a narcissist doesn't mean you have to live forever in their shadow. Whether your keeper is still in your life, or just a remnant of your past, you can free yourself from their shadow and create your own path of healing.

1. Learn all you can about narcissism

If you are someone who is just realizing that you are the victim of a childhood with a narcissist, you need to develop your knowledge before attempting to tackle the extremely complex task of dealing with a self-obsessed family member.

Having our database of knowledge accessible allows us to better deal with the complex emotions and conflicts that will continue to simmer due to our narcissistic upbringing. The more you know, the more you will be able to deflect any ongoing attacks they may inflict on you and the better you will be able to resolve the pain they have inflicted on you in the past.

The internet is full of great chapters and studies that will shed some light on the subject for you, and there is no shortage of family relations experts out there who can open some doors for you as well. The more you educate and find support, the more you will allow yourself to take the best action for you.

2. Start embracing your emotions

Often, one of the first steps in healing the harm done by narcissistic parents is to simply acknowledge and honor the feelings you have for that parent in the first place. In order for the self-obsessed to function continuously, they require those around them to bury their emotions deep inside. Taking them back and facing them means taking power away from the narcissist.

Sometimes our pain is mixed with anger and our guilt with compassion. It's also possible to become numb to your feelings over time, thanks to regular firing, cancellation, or just all-round marginalization.

Allow yourself to feel what you are feeling and don't judge yourself for it. Let the way you feel about your parents or the situation guide you in the direction of what you need most to heal. If that means ending family interactions that were once a part of your daily life, then that's what it means

3. Release the need to blame

Being a scapegoat from a self-obsessed parent can make you internalize an enormous amount of guilt and take the blame for something you had little or no control over. Narcissists are experts in deflection, but it's important to remember that we are all responsible for our own behavior.

4. Note the roles you play

Each family has roles and dynamics in which the various members play. In some families there is a scapegoat; while in others there is the golden child. Narcissistic parents retain control over their families by creating division between those families.

The best way to defend against this type of assault is to present a unified front, but it is something that requires cohesion and communication to be managed. Achieve mutual understanding and unity about the part you are playing and why, and try to strengthen each other rather than giving in to the divisive rhetoric your attacker uses to keep you "in your place."

5. Cultivate acceptance in your life

One of the hardest aspects of overcoming a self-centered parent is coming to the understanding that they will never change, no matter how much you want to or how sensibly you approach them.

Even when it seems like they're making great strides, it's often just a means of manipulation, and it's not long before the same old judgmental, vengeful, and critical opponent returns.

6. Let go of self-infliction

When we have grown up as impaired spectators of narcissists, we have a habit of picking up patterns that continue to inflict pain for days, weeks, and years. Those who have grown out of self-obsession are also those who are more prone to risky, counterproductive, and destructive behaviors that work to reinforce the limits their attacker projects on them.

Additionally, you exacerbate your trauma and create new destructive forces in your life that can seriously weaken your healing ability. If you want to overcome the abuse of a narcissistic parent, you must first stop harming yourself, but that requires looking inward and hugging that hurt and broken child with complete and accepting surrender.

7. Stick to your boundaries

Narcissists earn their power by constantly attacking borders. Even when we take off strongly against their onslaught, it is difficult to maintain that determination when our sense of self is tested endlessly. You are not respected by the narcissistic parent; you are object of objection - and this makes it essential to fight for your limits and reaffirm them on every available opportunity.

Borders protect us, so think about some protective borders that might be important to you. Consider what you want from them and which lines are absolutely unacceptable to cross. Just consider your feelings in this decision and leave everyone else out.

Really focus on the time it takes to create healthy boundaries that work just for you and your needs. Communicate these needs to your parents and let them know that, just like them, you no longer accept less than you deserve (even if that means limited contact).

Put it all together...

Warding off the toxic attacks of a narcissistic parent is never easy, no matter how old you are or how far you may wander. Self-obsessed parents harm their children in a number of alarming ways, and those effects follow their children as trauma and destructive coping mechanisms that destroy their well-being and quality of life in adulthood. Getting over a narcissistic education is difficult, but not impossible. You just need to foster some understanding and adopt the tactics and techniques that allow your authentic self to thrive.

DOUBLE BIND THEORY: TRAPPED BY THOSE WE LOVE MOST

"I want you to do what you want, but don't
do it because I told you."

This sentence is the epitome of the Double Bind Theory, or also called the Double Bind, a phenomenon that characterizes our interpersonal relationships and that is not only disconcerting, but can hurt us a lot, especially because it comes from the closest people, the most important, the ones we love the most.

What is the double bind theory?

The philosopher Karl Popper, famous for his "theory of forgery", one day sent a colleague the following postcard:

Dear MG:

Please send me this same postcard again after marking the empty rectangle to the left of my signature with a "yes" or any other sign if, for whatever reason, you think that when I receive the postcard, this space will be still empty.

Your friend, KR Popper

If this letter has nearly paralyzed your mind, don't worry, it's the normal result of confusion. A strategy often used by manipulators and that the anthropologist Gregory Bateson has cataloged as "Double Bind".

The double constraint occurs when:

The person has to do X, but they ask him to do Y as well, which conflicts with X.

In practice, it is when they ask us to do two opposite things, impossible to accomplish. They subject us to two conflicting imperatives, neither of which can be ignored. At this point we feel confused because we are faced with an insurmountable dilemma, because if we satisfy one of the requests, we cannot satisfy the other as well. Worse still, the situation is outlined in such a way that we are not even allowed to comment on how absurd the request is.

The spontaneity imposed

A typical example of a double bind situation is when a person asks us to show spontaneous behavior, but from the moment they make that request, our behavior ceases to be spontaneous. The necessary spontaneity inevitably leads to a paradoxical situation in which the mere fact of making the request makes it impossible to fulfill it spontaneously.

If she brings flowers, it won't be enough to satisfy the need for affection because we know it wasn't spontaneous behavior. In that case, we have put the other in a double bind situation. Make the decision you make, it will not be enough to satisfy our request because by doing it, we prevent its correct satisfaction.

A mother may blame the baby for being too listless and passive, so she is likely to say "move a little, don't be so dull".

In this case, there are only two possible solutions, both equally unsatisfactory: the child remains passive so the mother feels cheated, or she changes her behavior to satisfy her mother, but since this is not a natural and spontaneous attitude, she will consider his response as a sign of passivity, having limited himself to carrying out an order.

The conditions for producing the double constraint

A meaningful relationship between people. If the person is not important to us and has no emotional power, we will simply point out the absurdity of his request. Therefore, double bind situations usually become a weapon of manipulation of parents, partners or friends.

A mandate that prevents the "victim" from escaping the situation. It is the final touch to put the person with his back against the wall, also preventing him from expressing his disorientation and commenting on what is happening.

The dire consequences of growing up in a Double Bind environment

These antagonistic, mutually canceling requests block us simultaneously in three fields: thought, action and feeling. This constricting situation is highly harmful as it binds us hands and feet, preventing us from even expressing what we feel.

Paul Watzlawick systematized the double bind situations in everyday life, with the closest people, analyzing their impact on our personality.

• Deep personal insecurity

When we see that our perceptions of reality or of ourselves provoke the reproach of other people of vital importance to us, we feel inclined to distrust our senses.

If we grew up with parents telling us things like, "You have to be crazy to think like this," it's easy to understand the problem we're facing.

This description corresponds perfectly to the clinical picture of schizophrenia.

- **Immense sense of guilt**

The most terrible thing is that this guilt will add to the list of feelings we shouldn't have.

An example of this double bind situation is when parents assume that a well-bred child should be a happy child and turn their child's fleeting moments of sadness into a dull accusation of failure in their work as educators. Some parents may express that disappointment with phrases such as "after all we have done for you, you should feel happy and content."

In this way, the smallest sadness of the child turns into ingratitude and malice, creating the breeding ground for a tormented mind. He starts to think that something is wrong with him because he shouldn't feel sad.

- **Confusion of values**

Sometimes, people who are important to us demand behavioral norms that require and at the same time prevent certain actions.

This is the case of parents who ask their children to respect the rules, but also to dare. Or those who value money and think that every means is good for obtaining it, but who also encourage the child to be honest at all times.

The Double Bind Theory as a tool of manipulation and submission

It's a very powerful weapon for emotionally dominating someone because:

- He invalidates his views on the matter, dismissing his thoughts as "invalid" or "outright madness".
- Invalidate his feelings, making him feel guilty for them and, therefore, preventing him from expressing them, pain, be judged severely.
- Prevents action, forcing the person to remain in a no-way uncomfortable situation, the worst situation that can be found.

To get rid of this constraint and disarm the person who tries to turn us against the wall, it is enough to point out the contradiction.

TOXIC RELATIONSHIPS: 5 WAYS TO CURD THEM EVEN IN THE FAMILY

Nobody deserves to live in an emotionally toxic environment. Getting out of it is therefore not only necessary, but also absolutely vital. We all have toxic relationships within the family unit: these can make us feel very bad emotionally and make life difficult, if not impossible.

TOXIC RELATIONSHIPS IN THE FAMILY

The family is one of the typical scenarios in which the drama of "toxic relationships" is born and grows. Added to this is the fact that we cannot just get rid of them, as there will always be something that will unite us.

Ex-partners may exist, of course, but there is no ex-mother, ex-father, ex-brother, ex-grandfather, etc. In fact, we can end a relationship, but we cannot do the same with our relatives.

The family is imposed on us, we cannot choose and that means that, as much as we don't like it, we have to adapt. We are often subjected to rules within the family that make us feel suffocated.

This triggers a feeling of bondage, sorrow and makes us feel trapped, with no way out. Furthermore, the more important the "toxic relatives" are in the family, the more difficult it will be to get out and enforce our rights.

It is said that there are two types of families: rigid ones and flexible ones. In the first type, toxicity abounds, as it arises from the intense and irrational use of power.

This situation triggers a difficulty in relating to others and prevents us from freely expressing our feelings and opinions, establishing a dialogue or showing ourselves as we are.

These relatives are, without a doubt, emotional vampires. These are those people who subject us to the authority, envy and constant accusation of someone who, in reality, should take care of us more than anyone else in the world.

As we have said, the most logical and probable thing is not to be able to easily break the relationship, as a family bond cannot be lightly unraveled.

However, sometimes relationships become unsustainable and there is no other option but to escape the toxic environment.

HOW CAN YOU REACT?

According to the psychologist Laura Rojas Marcos, most conflicts arise from power struggles, the feeling of entitlement to others and the lack of limits.

What is the key to getting rid of the burden of a relative who hurts us with their actions and words? How to learn how to manage toxic relationships without making the situation worse?

1. Empathy: putting yourself in the other person's shoes

This does not mean that we must accommodate the wishes and needs of others, but be willing to understand what lies behind the words and gestures.

This means that "training empathy" implies being available to listen and consider what others have to say. This will help us to accept the possibility of not being able to reach an agreement because everyone has different needs.

In these cases, there must be a pact of respect for the disagreement, which will make coexistence easier. This means admitting that: "you want something that is not compatible with my wishes, let's accept it and move on".

2. Respect everyone's intimacy and personal space

Respecting the other means accepting the fact that the answer is "no", tolerating frustration even if it seems unfair. We cannot afford to think that "trust sucks", because the interference triggers great family conflicts.

In family relationships, aspects on which there is no agreement are taken for granted. If you arrive unannounced at your children's home or if you make a phone call at inconvenient times, you need to be prepared for an answer that we may not like and that traces the boundaries of the relationship.

3. Be respectful and stay calm

During family conversations, it is common to say the first thing that comes to mind. This happens because we don't measure our words and actions with education and respect.

Most of us are likely to have a close relative who thinks he can say anything and who considers his own ideas and opinions more important than those of others.

This is a source of conflict and it is therefore important to step away from the situation and set limits by discussing it calmly, noting that what the other says hurts us emotionally.

4. Be decisive and use magic words

Some family relationships are based on power plays. What you probably want is not power, but freedom of action and expression with no one to make your life difficult.

In these situations, we must stand up and be clear and decisive when we say "I can't", "I don't want" or "I don't agree". It is important to be confident, to act with determination and to use our decision-making power.

Even if we are in the family, it is still important to say "thank you" and "please" as this is how we express our consideration and courtesy, showing respect for the time and effort required for requests and favors.

5. Be patient

Being impatient makes us impulsive and unreasonable when we have to evaluate the circumstances and make a decision. For this reason, it is imperative to learn to wait and reflect before acting.

Sometimes it happens that we cannot get rid of the difficulties that add to the fatigue caused by "toxic family relationships". In these cases, it is essential to make decisions that break the family unit such as, for example, getting away from those people.

We must not forget that vampires and emotional predators exist in all contexts of our life, which means that we must learn to identify them and protect ourselves from them.

It is therefore very important to learn to control the intensity of feelings such as anger, which can trigger even more serious dramas.

In conclusion, to be able to better manage toxic relationships it is good to keep a clear mind and accurately evaluate the consequences of one's actions, taking into consideration the emotional and physical limits that must never be exceeded.

NARCISSISTIC PARENTS AND FAMILY ENTANGLEMENT: HOW TO FIND YOURSELF AND LET GO OF GUILT

We speak of dyadic or family entanglement when narcissistic parents go beyond the personal boundaries of a child (or other relative) through dysfunctional relationship patterns.

The roots of entanglement can be traced back to a collusive family system in which narcissistic parents pathologically identify with their children, passing this pattern down from generation to generation. The individuality of the child is totally denied except in relation to the will of the parent who considers him / her a mere extension of himself.

Within this dynamic, the boundaries are blurred and may even be considered undesirable; for this reason, the parent can come to perceive the child as his limb, discouraging any thought or emotion that tends towards autonomy or individuation.

The healthy boundaries in a relationship are those within which we can consider the other endowed with his own autonomy of thought, feeling and behavior. Narcissistic parents perceive free initiative as a danger to their obsessive control and dominance, therefore they tend to suppress and repress any attempt by the child to assert himself on the surrounding environment.

In a relationship of this type, the parent (one day the partner) will feel entitled to control the other, his thoughts, his feelings, opinions and behaviors.

*This dynamic determines in children a constant
and pathological sense of guilt.*

A narcissistic parent "trains" you to feel dependent on him / her: if you do not think, move, feel as he / she wants or do not fully share his will, his (always negative) opinions on others or do not agree on the fact that she / he is the best person in the world as well as the undisputed victim of age-old family wrongs from which you have to redeem him / her, if you do not fight his / her battles and therefore do not fully embrace him / her, he / she will abandon you or some mysterious catastrophe will occur and you will not survive.

You can't live without me. Well ... know that it is the exact opposite, but the narcissistic parent's fear of being alone, leads him / her to instinctively manipulate you and control you in order not to risk a degree of "separation" that can put him / her in front of himself / a and his inner poverty. The enmeshed parent reacts negatively if the son / daughter shows autonomy and convinces him / her that these initiatives are disrespectful, immoral, unjust, which will damage him / her, the relationship or the family balance, forcing the son / daughter to a life of implicit moral blackmail.

Children are no longer able to distinguish their thoughts and emotions from those of the narcissistic parents, they have to fight for the parent, think like him / her in order not to lose him / her and then act and absorb the emotional pain.

These children learn to **INTUIT AND ANTICIPATE THE NEEDS OF THE NARCISSIST PARENT** and to put their own aside. They train themselves to pathologically widen their psychological, emotional, physical and often sexual boundaries. The narcissistic parent is not afraid to admit that it is natural to claim that if he / she has suffered for something the son / daughter should back him / her, no ifs and buts. I worked with a person who was presented with the cost of all the diapers used by her mother, with the aim of blaming her and making her weigh how much effort she it had been to raise her. Sometimes the dynamics are clear, other times subtle, but the result doesn't change. It is blackmail, an unjust and parasitic relationship, which if not remedied can become the ground for future dysfunctional relationships in the couple.

The child who grows up in a narcissistic context is deprived of the right to exist (if not as a reflection of the parent) and to grow by developing his autonomy and personal talent. Her self-esteem is undermined by the potential blackmail of the controlling, entangled parent. This is why if mum or dad are angry, it means that I have to do something, that I am responsible for their state of mind. It is at this very moment that we begin to function as our parents' **THERMOMETERS AND MOOD STABILIZERS** and one day we would be used for the same function by parasitic friends or partners or simply put ourselves in that position to be abused, because abuse is the only form of love we know.

The enmeshed parent trains and educates the child to refer to others to have confirmation of his value, so in the future it is likely that this pattern of extreme self-sacrifice will turn into relational masochism. **Love CONDITIONED AND PACKAGED.** Too bad you will never get that love because the person you are serving, who you are flattering and who has deluded you into loving you... has no love for you. He is not able to prove it except for himself / herself and that vain hope that by role, maturity or age, he can finally realize that you are not his arm, but a person with your own identity. It's a bluff.... They control you because they have to, not because they love you. Or rather ... they love you in their own way and that is SICK.

TIPS FOR LIVING WITH A NARCISSIST AND INTRUSIVE PARENT

Learn to center yourself and rely only on yourself: start allowing yourself to feel how you are, what you feel and what you think. Make decisions based on your interests without being afraid of the emotional or behavioral reactions (real or imagined) of your narcissistic parent. If he gets angry, it's his problem. Do not accept gifts or favors when you are in trouble: this is the hardest part... it comes naturally to lean on a parent emotionally or on a practical level when we are in trouble.

The narcissistic parent, however, sees this as a flaw in the system that they can plug into and then blame you for help and torture you for life with guilt and blackmail. Establish boundaries: This means you stop feeling responsible for your parents' lives and their bad moods or discomfort. Learn to manage your spaces and expect them to be respected.

Subject vs Object: Start valuing yourself based on who you are and not how others judge you. The attribution of your value cannot depend on external judgment and what you get, but on who you are. If people love you "only if" then they don't love you but their need for an idealistic fetish.

Start a therapeutic path aimed at regenerating: every time you find yourself feeling conditioned emotions or acting in an automatic and self-destructive way, stop and try to understand what your inner child asks or needs to grow and emerge.

Pay attention to physical health: those who are used to putting themselves aside, tend to somatize because they are not in contact with their emotions and do not recognize their physical limits. Abused children stifle any emotion or physical need in function of various objectives often aimed at impressing themselves or others, in order to "shine" to the point of being seen. Remember that you will shine alone until you burn. They don't see you because they are blind, not because you don't shine..., but since they don't want it to be known... they convince you that you have something wrong with you.

Beware of Guilt: If you were raised by a narcissistic parent you will certainly feel compelled to snap whenever someone is in trouble or feel more responsible than you should. Observe and accept these feelings without necessarily acting on them.

If you grew up in a context like this, you can hypothesize a path aimed at awareness and regeneration.

CHAPTER 4 - HEALING

POST-TRAUMATIC STRESS DISORDER OR TRAUMA RELATED DISORDERS

What is Post Traumatic Stress Disorder

Post-Traumatic Stress Disorder (PTSD) is a severe clinical condition that in its chronic form only develops in a small fraction of trauma survivors. Recent research has shown that a traumatic experience is relatively common in the general population: the values range between 50-70% for women and 60% for men; 3.5% of the US population develop Post Traumatic Stress Disorder annually, while in the rest of the countries the figures are around 0.5-1.0%.

Symptoms of Post-Traumatic Stress Disorder

Following the traumatic event (eg earthquake, accident, physical, psychological or sexual violence), the most frequent symptoms of PTSD are:

Marked reactivity associated with the traumatic event:

- hypervigilance and strong alarm responses;
- concentration problems;
- sleep-related difficulties;

- marked physiological reactions to internal or external triggers and to the traumatic event.

Post-Traumatic Stress Disorder is a clinical picture that is often associated with other disorders among which we often find:

- Affective Disorders and Major Depression (50%)
- Panic Disorder and Social Phobia (20%)
- Dissociative Disorders in the Psychiatric Population (18.5%)
- Borderline Personality Disorder
- Substance abuse and addiction as memory management strategies (50% male, 30% female)

As regards the course of symptoms, about 60% of cases of Post-Traumatic Stress Disorder recover spontaneously in the first 12 months, without psychotherapeutic treatment, but still have post-traumatic symptoms that are often treated with drugs.

Causes of Post-Traumatic Stress Disorder

There is no safe hypothesis about the causes of Post-Traumatic Stress Disorder, however one of the most accredited hypotheses argues that following a serious psychological trauma, an imbalance of the nervous system seems to occur in the person, probably caused by changes in the neurotransmitters or adrenaline, cortisol, etc. This results in a blockage of the system and the information acquired at the moment of the event, including images, sounds, emotions and physical sensations, is preserved at the neurological level in its disturbing state. Therefore, this material continues to be triggered by a range of internal and external stimuli and expresses itself in the form of nightmares, flashbacks and intrusive thoughts.

As regards the risk factors for the development of Post-Traumatic Stress Disorder, some categories can be identified:

Pretraumatic variables:

- gender
- previous psychiatric disorders (anxiety and depression)
- possible genetic vulnerability
- low level of education (mildly)
- low socioeconomic status (mildly)
- married men (mildly)

Peritraumatic variables: (related to the event itself and to the severity of the trauma):

- level of perceived threat to life
- duration of the traumatic event
- unpredictability of the traumatic event

Post-traumatic variables:

- poor social support
- poor management skills

Psychopathological Constructs Related to Post Traumatic Stress Disorder

The most common "reasoning errors" in Post-Traumatic Stress Disorder are:

- dichotomous thinking (eg "If I can't get over this event, my sex life will be a complete failure", "That man was not fully capable of understanding and willing, so it's my fault")
- hypergeneralization (eg "I feel I must always protect myself from all men ...")
- selective abstraction (eg "During a terrorist attack on our base that lasted more than 3 hours, for about 2-3 minutes I felt confused and disoriented. This should not happen; it means that I am totally inadequate for the job I was given")

POST-TRAUMATIC STRESS DISORDER THERAPY

The two most effective forms of intervention to date are:

A) Pharmacological treatment

The acute symptomatology of PTSD is often characterized by severe levels of anxiety, terror and hopelessness accompanied by insomnia. Therefore, it is advisable to evaluate the need to associate the psychological intervention, especially in the early stages of treatment, with a pharmacological treatment that attenuates the intensity of the anxious symptoms by enhancing the psychotherapeutic action. From a pharmacological point of view, the antidepressants Selective Serotonin Inhibitors (SSRIs), in particular paroxetine and sertraline, have been shown to be useful in the alleviation of disturbing symptoms.

B) Psychotherapeutic treatment

After a thorough assessment of the situation and an accurate conceptualization of the case, the psychotherapeutic intervention for Post-Traumatic Stress Disorder is divided into several phases:

- Definition and management of "urgent" problems for the patient (eg impairment of daily function due to avoidances)
- Building a safe and collaborative therapeutic relationship for the patient
- Provide information about the disorder
- Stabilize the most disturbing symptoms with the use of symptom management techniques (e.g. relaxation techniques)
- Work on traumatic memories through exposure to painful memories
- Carry out a cognitive restructuring
- Preventing relapses

As for the therapeutic approaches, the two most effective and widespread are:

1. Trauma-focused cognitive-behavioral psychotherapy

We can group the cognitive-behavioral techniques that will be used in the different phases of treatment into three broad categories:

Exposure techniques.

They aim to familiarize the patient with feared situations in a safe climate by means of In vivo Exposure and Exposure to Memories in Imagination procedures.

In vivo exposures are carried out by agreeing with the patient feared situations and activities that can arouse the memory of the event, creating a hierarchy that goes from the easiest to the most difficult according to a USM score (subjective units of malaise) and leading the person to face them. one after the other.

Exposure in vivo is followed by exposure with the imagination of memories in order to help the person rethink what has happened, the emotions felt and correct the counterproductive beliefs. Exposure to memories occurs gradually allowing the patient, in the initial phase, to skip the most painful parts and to keep his eyes open; later, he will ask himself to close his eyes to make the images more vivid and to use a past tense in the story; in the end, he will be asked to speak in the present, to imagine the event from afar or as in a film.

2. Cognitive restructuring

Through cognitive restructuring, the patient with Post Traumatic Stress Disorder is helped to identify and modify the "errors of reasoning" and dysfunctional beliefs about themselves, others and the world that may pre-exist the trauma, but which often depend on influence of the latter on the patient's personal views on issues such as a sense of security, self-confidence, personal worth and trust in others.

3. Anxiety management techniques

For example, effective breathing and relaxation modalities and the identification of mental distraction strategies.

4. EMDR therapy

The EMDR approach (Eye Movement Desensitization and Reprocessing) focuses on the memory of disturbing traumatic experiences, particularly stressful from an emotional point of view, which may have contributed to the disorder and which lead people to therapy. One of the most important aspects in this type of therapy is the identification of life events that have been "traumatic". These events can be traumas due to accidents, griefs, earthquakes, natural disasters, but also interpersonal - relational traumas, such as the emotional traumas that are generated in the relationship with a dysfunctional attachment figure.

The EMDR goes to work on the memory of these events, in order to re-elaborate and reorganize them in memory, to ensure that these experiences lose the intense emotional component associated with them and that the cognitively dysfunctional learning acquires a more positive meaning. All this allows the patient to be able to use his "painful memories" in a constructive way, turning them into a resource.

Each individual has the innate ability to process traumatic events, but in some people, in particularly serious situations, this ability is blocked. EMDR using bilateral stimulation, i.e. eye movements, is able to restart the processing capacity. EMDR is supported by a lot of scientific research and is recognized as a treatment of choice for Post-Traumatic Stress Disorder: specifically, for events that have resulted in life-threatening or threatening the person's integrity, the treatment is recognized as among the most effective.

New approaches to Post Traumatic Stress Disorder therapy we use:

METACOGNITIVE THERAPY (MCT)

Metacognitive Therapy is based on the assumption that the natural processing process of traumatic material is hindered by specific methods of processing information that alter the normal processing activity of traumatic memories, intrusive thoughts and emotions, frequent after a traumatic event. On the basis of this hypothesis, a therapeutic intervention is aimed at modifying thought processes such as brooding, attention strategies focused on the event that allow an elaboration of traumatic memories. From the first efficacy studies, Metacognitive Therapy appears to be a short-term treatment for Post-Traumatic Stress Disorder that produces high rates of reduction of specific symptoms and improvement in quality of life.

SENSOMOTOR THERAPY

Sensomotor Therapy refers to body psychotherapy as a basis for therapeutic skills and integrates techniques of psychodynamic psychotherapy, cognitive-behavioral therapy, with neuroscience. Through awareness "on the body" patients with PTSD learn to work within a "safe emotional space" so that the patterns of emotional activation are more regulated within a range, where it would be possible to work maintaining a balanced personal functioning. Once this has been achieved, traumatic memories can be treated. Patients are taught the concept of "modulation" in order to implement the ability to "transition" from negative emotional states to positive emotional states, using bodily experiences to integrate them with the aspect of awareness: for example, during an active phase, a client may be asked to "find a place in his body where he feels calm or neutral."

DURATION AND TIMING OF THE TREATMENT OF POST-TRAUMATIC STRESS DISORDER

It is impossible to accurately define the duration of treatment for Post-Traumatic Stress Disorder since there are many factors that influence it, among these we include: precocity of the intervention, psychopathological complexity, presence / absence of social support, personality of the patient. Therefore, the duration of a treatment varies from a few sessions to 8/12 months. The more complex the clinical picture, the longer will be the time to complete the treatment steps, even if the format and general structure remain similar.

DIFFICULTY IN MANAGING TRAUMATIC EXPERIENCES

If you've been through a traumatic experience, you may be struggling with upsetting emotions, frightening memories, and a sense of constant danger that you can't get rid of; or conversely, you may feel "disconnected", numb and unable to trust others. An emotional and psychological trauma is the result of extraordinary stressful events, which shatter the sense of personal security, making you feel helpless and vulnerable in a dangerous world. Traumatic experiences often pose a threat to life or safety, but any situation in which we feel overwhelmed and alone can be traumatic, even if it does not involve physical harm. Emotional and psychological trauma can be caused by a single event, such as a serious accident, natural disaster, or violence, but it can also result from the continuity of stressful events such as living in a neighborhood with a high crime rate or when you face a disease such as cancer.

Not all potentially traumatic events, however, involve permanent emotional and psychological damage, much also depends on the subjective response to the trauma and some personal vulnerability factors. A number of risk factors make people susceptible to emotional and psychological trauma, for example if they are already under a heavy load of stress, if they have recently suffered major losses or if they have suffered trauma before, for example in childhood. When childhood trauma is not resolved, in fact, the deep sense of fear and helplessness is carried over into adulthood, often laying the foundations for further trauma. Following a traumatic event, most people experience a wide range of physical and emotional reactions, these are normal reactions to abnormal events.

The most common emotional symptoms following trauma are: shock, rejection, disbelief, confusion, difficulty concentrating, anger, irritability, mood swings, despair, anxiety and fear, social withdrawal, shame and guilt. On a physical level, on the other hand, you can often have nightmares, insomnia, nervousness or agitation, flashbacks, muscle tension and tachycardia.

It can be important to seek the help of a psychologist when, despite the fact that some time has already passed, you still have terrifying memories, nightmares, flashbacks, you are avoiding more and more things that remind you of the trauma, you are isolating yourself and you begin to have problems at work and personal level, use alcohol or drugs to feel better or when you suffer from Post-Traumatic Stress Disorder (PTSD); the latter is the most severe form of response to emotional and psychological trauma. Its main symptoms are intrusive memories and flashbacks, avoidance of situations that recall the traumatic event and the experience of a constant state of "red alert".

To overcome a psychological and emotional trauma it is important to give yourself time, it is necessary to face and resolve the sometimes-unbearable feelings and memories that, for a long time, have been avoided. It is important to be patient and not to force the pace of healing in order to give yourself the opportunity to express what you are feeling and to mourn the losses.

TOXIC EMOTIONS PREVENT US FROM BEING HAPPY

Although fears or anxiety are emotions that, in the right dose, help us in survival, when they are present in excess, they are harmful. It is therefore important to learn to control them

We are aware that in the field of psychology and personal growth, the word "toxicity" is perhaps overused. For example, we often hear about toxic people or toxic behaviors. This changes when we talk about toxic emotions. Here we refer to emotions that harm or limit our psychological well-being and happiness.

Sometimes, in fact, some concepts find their best translation in these terms borrowed from other contexts.

In reality, there are no "toxic" people. There are people who, more simply, are unable to build relationships that are healthy, satisfying or based on mutual respect.

The word "toxic" therefore has no scientific value, but rather illustrates a dysfunctional behavior that causes discomfort, pain or unhappiness.

Today in our space we talk about this: the emotions that most threaten the emotional balance and in so doing, the possibility of building and leading a happier and more satisfying life.

1. Shame

It is said that over the years shame is lost, but there are those who intensify it to surprising levels, applying it to almost every area of their life.

Shame manifests itself in many ways. There is the shame of showing ourselves as we are, of wearing certain clothes, of asking others, of showing ourselves vulnerable, of trusting, of talking to the people who most attract us ...

It is clear that in social interactions and in daily life there are definite limits, barriers that we never cross for reasons of morality, convention or decorum.

However, in the area of personal growth, one thing must be clear: shame suffocates our true identity and our self-realization.

The feeling of shame has to do with fear and insecurity. It is therefore never too much to deepen the knowledge of ourselves, especially of what we do not accept or of the aspects of our personality on which it is more painful to work.

2. Anxiety: one of the most dangerous toxic emotions

Anxiety is toxic when it crosses the physiological threshold that gives us the motivation, the urge to demand more from ourselves.

When we come to perceive a continuous state of threat, stress or corrosive anxiety, we speak of toxicity, that is, a negative emotion capable of overwhelming us.

Chronic anxiety, far from stimulating us to improve, discourages, exhausts and deprives us of concentration.

3. Anguish, subtle among toxic emotions

Anguish is a time bomb: multiple negative dimensions are compressed in it: fear, feeling of threat, negativity, uncertainty, low resistance to frustration, pain.

No one can live eternally immersed in anguish. It is a way to die while staying alive, to completely deny ourselves the possibility of being happy and fulfilling ourselves as people.

4. Eternal dissatisfaction

In some circumstances, dissatisfaction acts as a powerful engine that pushes us to change, to overcome ourselves, to improve.

When dissatisfaction becomes chronic and unjustified, however, malaise and apathy invade everything.

Thus, little by little we lose the desire to do things, the fortitude, the smile and the motivation.

Beware of chronic dissatisfaction - this is often likely to be one of the symptoms of depression.

5. Envy

To envy others is not correct and not even healthy. Experiencing this feeling or emotion throughout our life has the only effect of bringing our self-esteem very low.

Envy leads along the path of suffering. Desiring for ourselves qualities, objects or dimensions that do not belong to us or that we are unable to obtain is painful and not useful for our psychological well-being.

Not being able to rejoice in the successes of others, to respect or appreciate what others are or have, says a lot about us.

We need to be able to rejoice in our successes, love each other and also appreciate what others are achieving.

6. Constant fear

If we wanted to give a simple definition of happiness, we could say: absence of fear.

We know that fears have a specific task: they help us survive; they alert us when we take a risk.

But when we get to the point where everything scares us, where the feeling dominates us that every action, we take will turn out badly, every change is negative and we feel criticized, abandoned or persecuted, we are boycotting our happiness.

7. Frustration

A "healthy" frustration stimulates change, overcoming our limits. Toxic frustration strands us on the beach of fears, broken dreams and surrender.

It cannot be ignored that frustration feeds on our failures, disappointments, unfulfilled dreams and unfulfilled goals.

Before becoming a grudge person, therefore, let's practice learning from our mistakes and failures to look forward, to apply new strategies, to regain control of our lives and be successful in the fields that are most important to us.

We have therefore seen that these emotions, which we all experience to some extent, can have a positive aspect, if we can keep them under control.

When they are the ones who hold the reins of our life and we ourselves make them sit in the palace of our mind without reacting, they will become toxic emotions ...

THE INNER CRITICAL VOICE (HOW TO RECOGNIZE IT AND LET IT GO)

Have you ever heard that voice critically telling you that you're not doing enough? Or that it lets you believe that you are not competent in the work you do ... that you could disappoint the people you love ...

That critical voice that usually makes it seem real and obvious as if they were real, situations that could happen; telling you "Oh! why did you say that? " ... and then lingers on that insignificant mistake for hours, even days. It is also the voice that constantly confronts you, reminding you that your goals seem far from your reach.

In some moments it is easy for negative thoughts to arise, for example when we are doing something important or new (facing a job interview, going on a first date). However, persistence, frequency and duration of such thoughts are the criteria for understanding whether they are part of the physiological and sporadic apprehension of a new challenge or if, instead, they are within a complex system of emotions and rigid attitudes towards oneself (and towards the others), almost audible, like the sound of a (critical) voice constantly speaking in a devaluing way (You haven't done enough! You will also ruin this relationship...).

What the inner critical voice is made of

The critical voice (or the inner critic) is defined as a system of evaluative and hostile thoughts towards oneself and others, well integrated with one's personal history. The critical voice is experienced as something external from which, however, one cannot free oneself. More technically, "internal criticism or self-criticism is represented by a severe and normative voice that interferes with the process of the individual's immediate experience".

The inner critical voice, far from being a "motivator" useful to push us further and further, is at the origin of many non-functional and unhealthy behaviors, representing a kind of enemy of personal growth, self-realization and well-being.

In fact, self-criticism and perfectionism are different from ambition, although sometimes they get confused. Without forgetting that this attitude towards oneself is an essential characteristic of some psychological disorders (including depressive disorder, eating disorder, obsessive-compulsive personality disorder).

For many people, self-criticism is seen as the source of personal success. On the contrary, studies show that this way of approaching oneself is more often connected with distrust, anxiety, dependence on the judgment of others and the onset of bad habits.

*"Understanding the difference between
healthy effort and perfectionism is key to
spreading the shield and getting your life back.
Research shows that perfectionism hinders
success. In fact, it is often the path to
depression, anxiety, addiction and life paralysis"*

(Brené Brown, The Gifts of Imperfection)

AN EXERCISE IN THE IMAGINATION

Now imagine that your inner critic is a close friend and imagine having lunch with him / her or going for a walk. So, imagine that all afternoon, this person is standing there judging you in a reproachful tone. Criticising your clothing, what you ordered for lunch, your plans for the weekend, and what you said to your boss.

Can you imagine how you will feel at the end of the day? Maybe you will feel unworthy, inadequate, disappointed, maybe angry, you certainly won't feel motivated or satisfied. You probably won't want to spend time with this over-critical friend very soon.

Likewise, if you feel that you are giving your inner critical voice a lot of space by allowing it to stay as long as it wishes, you can begin to recognize when you tell yourself things you would never tell others ...

... And let it go

WHAT IS SOCIAL PHOBIA?

Social phobia is the fear or anxiety of situations that involve the possibility of being criticized, judged, or being the center of attention. In fact, the person often avoids social interactions. These situations include social interactions in which new people meet, parties, situations in which the individual can find himself the center of attention.

Other feared situations can be:

- Using public restrooms
- Calling people on the phone
- Writing or working in the presence of other people
- Being the center of attention
- ing to people you are not familiar with
- Being criticized
- Talking to 'important' or authoritative people
- Going on a date
- Talking in class or at a meeting
- Eating or drinking in public
- Taking exams or tests
- Being called to class for questioning

The person's fear is to be negatively evaluated by others, to do something embarrassing, to be humiliated and rejected, or to offend other people.

Being watched or at the center of attention can be torture

What are the symptoms of social phobia disorder?

Social phobia disorder is a condition of subjective suffering characterized by fear and restlessness, usually associated with somatic symptoms (tremors, flushing, tachycardia, dyspnoea, dizziness, etc.) and with marked and persistent fear of a social situation, expected or from face, in which you are exposed to evaluation by others. The main characteristics of the disorder are the following:

- fear and anxiety of one or more social situations in which the person is exposed to the possible judgment of others: eg. meeting unknown people, holding a conversation, being observed while eating, giving a public speech
- the person is afraid of acting or showing anxiety symptoms and that, therefore, will be negatively evaluated by others
- fears situations that cause anxiety and fear, and are therefore often avoided
- the fear and anxiety are disproportionate, and the person is aware of them
- the disorder causes significant discomfort or impairment of the person's performance in the various areas of his life (work, social, leisure)

Social phobia is not introversion!

Social phobia must be distinguished from introversion: in the case of the introverted person, we are simply in the presence of choices suggested by a personal hierarchy of preferences for different activities; in the case of social fears we are in the presence of a renunciation of desired social activities, but made intolerable by the presence of too high levels of tension and anxiety.

The concerns of social phobia

Most of the time these are widespread fears, ie the subject fears more than one situation; more rarely, anxiety is limited and can be accompanied by multiple pictures of psychophysiological disorders that occur, or that the subject fears may arise, in specific contexts and thus induce the systematic avoidance of some significant social situations.

The central concern of the person with social anxiety is being judged to be anxious, weak, crazy, stupid, boring, unpleasant; fears that, in a relational context, he will act or appear inadequate or that he will show anxiety symptoms such as blushing, shaking, sweating, stumbling over words and that for this he will be negatively evaluated by others. It is common to self-medicate with substances in order to cope with feared situations and manage unpleasant physical sensations (e.g. drinking alcohol at a party to decrease the level of anxiety).

Social phobia

There are often very negative expectations about the judgment and intentions of others

Anticipatory anxiety

In addition to the anxiety or fear associated with the dreaded situation, anticipatory anxiety is common, i.e. anxiety that begins days or weeks before the moment in which that situation will have to be faced. This can trigger a vicious circle in which anticipatory anxiety causes such a state of anxiety that the person truly has a really poor or embarrassing performance.

For example, a person might arrive at a job interview tense, sweaty, struggling to express himself, uncertain and stammering. Thus a 'self-fulfilling prophecy' occurs: the fear of poor performance at the interview really causes poor performance. So, if he has to interview again, he'll be even more anxious.

How can I tell if I have social phobia?

Only an experienced psychotherapist can confidently diagnose a social phobia disorder.

If you are afraid of exposing yourself and being criticized, if you fear and / or avoid social situations and this causes you significant discomfort or limits your performance in certain areas of your life (e.g., in work and private life) you should seek professional advice.

At ITC we use comprehensive psychological assessments by integrating information from interviews, psychological tests and psychophysiological observations.

Associated problems

Social phobia is often associated with other anxiety disorders, depressive disorders or substance use disorder. The coexistence of depression is high, especially in the older adult population and can be the result of chronic isolation, while the substances can be used as self-medication.

Although self-criticism has been a topic of great interest in the psychotherapy literature for several decades, the construction of explanatory models and research into what generates self-criticism has been very limited. An exception has been attachment theories, which have developed a model that links the uncompromising criticism of oneself to affective relationships with normative attachment figures, not emotionally accessible, poorly attuned to the needs of the child and prone to devaluation. The hypothesis is that the emotional style of the relationship can become the model by which one will later turn to oneself.

As a therapist, I work with many competent and very talented people. While these qualities of theirs seem very clear to me, they have difficulty seeing them in themselves. They are in fact very busy bringing a hyper-focus onto frailties and minor defects. This prevents them from maintaining a broader perspective that recognizes their progress and accepts its limitations.

How to give that voice some relaxation and calm?

Following the suggestions of Sharon Salzberg, pioneer of Mindfulness in the USA and founder of the Insight Meditation Society with Joseph Goldstein, it is useful, first of all, to be able to stop and notice this voice within oneself. Then, after noticing it, observing it carefully, you can try to give it a name and a wardrobe, offer it a tea and a chance to rest... It must be really tired, with its great brooding over all those negative thoughts" (Sharon Salzberg).

THE 5 STEPS TO HEALING FROM NARCISSISTIC ABUSE

When one thinks of trauma, one usually tends to imagine isolated events such as natural disasters or car accidents.

But trauma can take many forms.

Narcissistic abuse is a form of trauma that devastates the soul, as it slowly builds up like an avalanche.

In many cases, it affects one's identity and mental health on a very deep level and over several years.

That is why the stages of healing after narcissistic abuse are an ongoing process, not an instant event.

Healing from complex trauma such as narcissistic abuse requires a very different approach than recovering from isolated traumatic events.

It's not easy or quick, but you'll come out of it more dignified, strong, and kind than it ever was before the abuse.

Because healing from narcissistic abuse is different

In fact, the complex trauma of narcissistic abuse is similar to living under siege in a state of war (psychological fighting and torture) and blocking (emotional, spiritual, and even physical isolation) for many years.

Narcissistic abuse trauma is the frequent result of trying to have a healthy and functional relationship with a person with personality disorders over a long period of time.

During the relationship with a narcissist, cognitive dissonance and a devastating traumatic bond develops in the victim due to the strategic use of psychological manipulation techniques, such as silent treatment.

Now: if the narcissist is always to be the victim, it means that the culprit must always be someone else.

Yes, this is your role: you are the antagonist and he is the protagonist of the hypothetical film that takes place in his head.

All of this has an impact on how you see yourself and everyone around you.

Whenever one experiences another cycle of emotional abuse with the narcissist, there is a very precious moment, which we can define as THE TIME OF CHOICE.

This is where we have the opportunity to change the vicious circle that has become a habitual and automatic pattern in our life.

And it's certainly hard to stop and think about this when you're in constant fight-or-flight mode during narcissistic abuse.

But the choices we make now are not just about our future, but also about the future of our children, our friendships, our workplace, our life.

In moments of abuse and emotional devastation - which are inevitable within a relationship with a narcissist - we just want to feel better about ourselves, stop the pain, and get things back to normal.

It is nearly impossible to think rationally in moments of emotional abuse.

But, even in moments of unbearable anguish, there is that split second when your mind tells you, "See, we knew it was going to happen. I don't know why you don't listen to me."

These are the times when you can choose and break the cycle of abuse.

RECOVERY FROM NARCISSISTIC ABUSE IS A MARATHON, NOT A SPRINT.

A complex trauma from narcissistic abuse takes a long time to develop and it is naive, therefore, to believe that recovery from narcissistic abuse can be instantaneous.

The narcissist has spent years slowly destroying your sense of self and your spirit.

Consequently, trauma healing should be an ongoing process. It is therefore essential to work through the PHASES OF RECOVERY FROM TRAUMA. The effects of a complex narcissistic abuse trauma will follow you wherever you go - as you seek a new job, seek new friends, try to rebuild lost relationships, and try to develop an identity again.

And this new identity of yours will never be the same again.

You probably already know the five stages of grief.

The stages of recovery from narcissistic abuse are very similar.

1. STABILIZATION. PHASE OF NO CONTACT

This first phase of recovery from narcissistic abuse is the most important, but it is also the most difficult.

The 'No Contact' is finally put in place by the narcissist and you are not sure if you have made the right decision, precisely because you are still under the effect of the hyperstimulation derived from narcissistic abuse.

What you need now is support and reassurance.

You have been subjected to a level of stress and abuse for so long that experiencing security and calm will feel strange, if not wrong.

You are still vulnerable and are afraid of how the narcissist will respond to everything you think or do.

2. PHASE OF STANDING UP

This is the time you start recovering.

Your energy begins to return after the narcissist has drained it for so long.

The only way to counter this is to find an emotionally available attachment figure after starting No Contact.

It could be a friend, a family member, a therapist, anyone who can protect and support you ... at least during the first few months of No Contact.

This is the stage where a good narcissistic abuse recovery program can make a difference.

3. THE STAGE OF WITHDRAWAL

The third of the key stages in healing after narcissistic abuse is a very delicate one.

One begins to rebuild one's identity, but the past tends to get in the way. You may start to give the narcissist too much credit and think "we treated each other badly" or "he was abused too."

Now that you begin to feel confident in yourself and your decisions, you may feel able to address the narcissist casually ... maybe he's changed ...

No: he hasn't changed.

During this phase, you will have to deal with abstinence from the biochemical addiction that has formed after repeated cycles of abuse.

When you are in withdrawal, your mind will tell you all sorts of things to get you back in touch with it so that you can have a dopamine rush. He will tell you that things can go back to the way they were before, before the abuse started in full force.

For a while, this idea will seem feasible to you as your brain clings to fragile memories, leaving you with a yearning. You will convince yourself that you have overreacted to everything.

At the very least, you may find yourself looking for an explanation.

Stop: Reopening contact with the narcissist will set you back in your recovery or, worse, it will send you right back into the cycle of abuse.

4. THE PHASE OF OBJECTIVE ANALYSIS

At this point, in healing from narcissistic abuse, one can objectively look at one's past without feeling overwhelmed by emotions such as anger or regret.

You have spent a lot of time looking inside yourself and identifying the emotional triggers left behind by narcissistic abuse.

You are now ready to move on.

If you've made it this far, your life is now finally a blank canvas on which to paint a beautiful watercolor of your future.

5. STAGE OF ACCEPTANCE

At this stage, you can finally see things clearly as they are.

Know your abilities and limitations, not the ones the narcissist has instilled in you.

At this point, you know how to develop healthy relationships and have the courage to take action if someone tries to treat you badly.

It is absolutely critical to go through the five stages of trauma recovery while recovering from narcissistic abuse.

It is necessary to analyze how the trauma developed in order to unravel it definitively.

www.ingramcontent.com/pod-product-compliance
Lightning Source LLC
Chambersburg PA
CBHW062108040426
42336CB00042B/2665